Gluten Free College Student Cookbook

201

Gluten Free Recipes
for the College Student

A Gluten Free Success Publication

By Joanne Bradley

Notice

This book is intended as a culinary reference only. Dietary suggestions contained in this work may not be appropriate for all individuals, and readers should consult with a physician before commencing any dietary program. The information given here is designed to help you make informed decisions. The publisher and author hold no responsibility in how this information is put to use. Mention of specific companies, organizations or authorities in this book does not imply endorsement by the publisher, nor imply that they endorse this book.

ISBN-10: 1442179805

EAN-13: 9781442179806

Printed in the United States of America

by Gluten Free Success Publications
Lockport, New York 14095
www.gfcfsuccess.com

Quick Content Guide...

Recipes at a Glance...

Introduction

Finally, a cookbook just for you,
the gluten free college student.

Gluten Free College Student Cookbook

Welcome to 201 ways to make your gluten free college dining a safe and tasty experience!

These recipes are uniquely designed to be:

- ◆ Low-cook meals and snacks that use common ingredients in common sizes easily found in dorm refrigerators across the country.

- ◆ Economical as possible for the college student's budget.

- ◆ Easy to find ingredients that are available on or near college campuses.

- ◆ Made using the microwave, rice cooker, stove top, or toaster oven rather than a full kitchen.

- ◆ Effortless for allergen substitutions.

- ◆ Vegan and vegetarian friendly with soy, gluten free grains, or bean substitutions.

- ◆ Healthier choices than processed or junk foods.

There is no denying that the college experience can be a challenge to the average student, not to mention those on a gluten free diet. You may think... Will I be able to find gluten free foods to eat? Will my grades suffer from being ill all the time? Or even worse, will my social life be as a food wallflower, permanently alienated from my peers?

No, no and NO!

With this book, you will quickly discover how easy it is to make foods to take with you in a knap sack or share at a dorm event. Even your late night snacks will be better than what other students are eating. Be prepared to be the most popular person in your dorm – you will be the one with all the good food!

Your first year away from the comfort of a gluten free kitchen might be traumatic at first. There will be a learning curve and that is one of the reasons I wrote this book for you. I have worked with college students for many years in professional foodservice, preparing food for a whole spectrum of tastes and food desires. During that time, I learned how difficult it was to serve foods gluten free. And then I learned about it first hand when I was diagnosed with multiple food intolerances, including gluten and dairy.

So this book is a personal journey as well as a guide for gluten free persons of all ages. I set aside my gourmet leanings and thought about everyday foods, done fast and tasty. With a special insight into what college students crave on a daily basis, I tailored the recipes to this special situation. Lack of cooking equipment, space constraints, and the logistics of grocery shopping on campus should not hinder a healthy gluten free lifestyle.

The Tips and Tidbits section is devoted to bringing a beginning cook up to speed quickly. Learning how to do basic cooking skills like measure liquids and solids, dice vegetables, brown meat, and boil water can be time consuming at first, but quickly turns into preparing food on "auto pilot." Cooking is a learning experience. You may start out with a basic need to feed yourself but then become excited to learn a range of kitchen skills as you master the creation of gluten free meals.

I personally think of recipes as guidelines, not written in stone. I encourage you to explore the world of cooking as fun and adventuresome. I have found that most mistakes are still edible, and you learn from the experience. And that is what college (and life) are all about.

Enjoy using this book and I hope it is of true service to you in your college years and beyond.

Joanne Bradley

June 2009

Tips and Tidbits

About Cooking on Campus

Gluten Free College Student Cookbook

About Being on the Gluten Free Diet

The gluten free and dairy free recipes in this book have been written for people medically diagnosed with gluten intolerance that can lead to many autoimmune diseases. It is not a fad diet but a medically prescribed diet. Those on the gluten free diet have to be very vigilant and exacting when it comes to not consuming gluten in any form.

That being said, the gluten free diet is now being marketed as a lifestyle and wellness diet. Gluten intolerance is a spectrum of issues that affect many people, usually without their knowledge. For example, Celiac disease is statistically under-diagnosed by as much as 97% of people who have it. Other researchers have reported that the spectrum of gluten intolerance (not just Celiac disease) may reach up to 3 or 4 percent of the American population. At this writing, these numbers are not confirmed scientifically, and we will have to wait for future studies to illuminate the depth of gluten intolerance in the general population.

If you feel better when you don't eat wheat or gluten, and stop eating it, you may prevent an accurate medical diagnosis. Talk to your medical professional first about going on the gluten free diet. As with any food plan, your physician's expertise should partner with you in a healthy diet.

One of the positive outcomes of eating gluten free is the great health benefits of eating fresh, non-processed foods. Since wheat is often an ingredient in processed meats, prepared mixes and foods, when you are on the gluten free diet you begin to eat healthier foods in general. This principle can be applied to all people – fresh food is best!

This cookbook is about making good food while being a college student. It emphasizes gluten and dairy free recipes that can be used by all students as part of their balanced diet.

About the Recipes

When starting to use any cookbook, there are often guidelines to make the best use of the recipes in the book. Gluten free cooking and baking can be even more involved. So please read this section before using the recipes. It contains information that applies to all of the recipes and will help you understand what the instructions mean or help you choose ingredients. As always, have fun.

The abbreviation for gluten free used throughout the book is "**GF.**" The abbreviation for gluten free and casein free is "**GF/CF.**"

> All ingredients should be **gluten free** when you purchase them. Please remember to read the labels before buying. Items are not specifically marked gluten free in the recipes as all ingredients should be. As a reminder, foods highlighted in **bold** are often contaminated with gluten. **Always use products that are safe for your specific diet.** If you are very new to the diet, a simple reference guide to the gluten free diet is included at the end of the recipe section.

This book assumes that you have a working knowledge of the gluten free diet and your individual food intolerances/allergies. Many quality books exist to get people started on the gluten free diet. This cookbook focuses on common gluten free challenges with foods for a college campus. If you are unsure of what to eat, please check your library or bookstore for a more complete reference on the gluten free lifestyle.

All of the recipes in this book are easy to substitute with other foods for various allergies or taste preferences. For example – you can use different vegetables for the ones listed, substitute ground turkey in place of ground beef, or use any sweetener instead of sugar. View these recipes as *guidelines* to your own personal expression. They are very simple and very forgiving. Have fun and follow your own food tolerances.

Cheeses and other dairy foods are presented with the **casein free** version first, and the dairy version second. If you can eat dairy products, you will find it very easy to substitute your favorite cheeses or milk. Soy cheeses melt at very high heats compared to dairy cheese and are added sooner in the cooking process. It is specified in the recipe when to add the dairy cheese if it will make a difference in the end product.

Dairy free cheeses vary widely. The recipes in this book were tested with a *meltable* **soy cheese** that comes in several flavors. Other dairy free cheeses may work as well, or not! You may have to experiment with them to achieve a good result.

A common measurement in this book is for 1 oz. (ounce) of cheese. This is equivalent to about 1/8 cup of shredded cheese. An easy way to measure out an ounce is to look at the total weight of the package (for example 8 ounces) and visually divide the block of cheese into 8 sections. Cut off one section for one ounce. You can cut all sections and store in a reclosable bag for convenience if it makes it easier for you. Or, crumble cheese into a measuring cup to equal 1/8 cup.

Cutting a stick of margarine or butter into tablespoons is similar to cutting a block of cheese. Each tablespoon section is marked on the outer wrapping paper. A teaspoon of margarine or butter is *one-third* of a tablespoon. Visually divide the tablespoon section into 3, and cut off one teaspoon. Cream cheese in a block can be measured in the same way.

Dry pasta is often listed in ounces (oz). You probably don't have a scale in your room so you can use the same estimation method as above. A package of pasta is usually 16 ounces. So for 2 ounces, visually divide the total amount into 8 sections. You will soon be able to estimate 2 ounces of pasta with confidence.

Seasoning food is a skill, but only you can tell if it tastes good to you. Start with ¼ teaspoon of an unfamiliar spice or herb and add seasoning in small increments. Please use your creative side to experiment with different tastes and spices. It's what makes good food into great food!

The recipes are also marked for the type of **appliances** they can be cooked with. You will see a heading on each recipe that looks like this...

Rice Cooker, Stovetop, Microwave

When cooking with different appliances, the time it takes to cook may differ widely. Microwave wattage will make a difference in the timing. The type of pans or rice cooker you use will change the length of time to the desired result. **Please keep in mind the guidelines in the recipes should never overshadow your own common sense about cooking.** Be prepared to be flexible should it take more or less time to cook the foods to how you like them done.

Vegan and vegetarian friendly recipes are marked as such in the heading. *Friendly* means that vegan ingredients can easily be substituted for those listed. It does not mean that the recipe as written is vegan or vegetarian, only that it can become so with commonly used vegan ingredients. Often tofu is listed as the alternative, but you can use your vegan imagination to substitute proteins in the recipes. It is more of a marker of where to substitute rather than an absolute recommendation.

The **Nutrition Information** listed after each recipe can help you maintain a healthy weight at college. The style of the recipes is to provide quality nutrition and taste without excess fats or calories. You may want to substitute lower calorie or lower fat products for those listed. Although not tested with the lower versions, most recipes will come out well with many "light" products.

A note about the freshman five, ten or fifteen...

Eating from just one group of foods will have a tendency to put on weight, especially a diet focused on carbohydrates. Pasta, noodles, and baked goods are quick and easy in a college student's lifestyle. However, it will show up eventually as extra poundage. Eating fresh fruits and vegetables is more important than the convenience of high starch foods. Fresh produce provides the "brain food" that every student needs.

The recipes in this book are skewed toward easy carbohydrate and protein foods that are typically not gluten free in a college setting. They complete a balanced diet but are not a complete diet in themselves. In other words, balance out bowls of noodles or pasta with fresh foods. Gluten free fresh fruits, vegetables and salad bars are commonly available in cafeterias and food outlets all over campus. So feast on these in addition to selecting recipes from this book for a well balanced diet.

Help is available on most campuses for learning about a healthy diet. Many universities have dieticians on staff through the medical facilities or wellness centers on campus. There may also be a dietician available through the food service. These benefits are usually free to enrolled students, so don't be shy about asking for this service.

Portion size is a hot topic right now. For the purposes of this book, a portion is smaller than restaurant servings you may be familiar with. A restaurant portion is oversized and will put on oversized weight. The number of portions in the recipe is listed and you can determine what your serving size should be. Many recipes can be considered "side dishes," but if eaten as a main meal, a double portion may be appropriate. If you are very active or an athlete, a double portion may not be enough. Use the information given in the recipes as a guideline for your own good health.

Many of the recipes include additional tips for **Creative Cooking**. These are suggestions on how to vary or add to the recipe so that it becomes your own creation. If you are ready to experiment and refine your food to your own tastes, these suggestions are for you!

Go Ahead…

Dive In !

Cooking Techniques

Cooking is simple once you know a few simple methods. Great chefs use the same techniques that are available to you. The difference is that they have practiced and mastered their craft. Understanding a few basic skills can lead you to some mighty fine food, so pay attention!

Basic techniques include: baking, roasting, broiling, grilling, searing, braising, steaming, sautéing, boiling and simmering. One at a time, we will simplify these for the beginning cook.

Baking uses dry heat and is done in the oven. The most common types of baked foods include breads, cakes, pies, muffins, vegetables, meats, and casseroles. Practically any type of food can be baked including vegetables and fruits.

Roasting is a slow-method of cooking food and involves the use of dry heat. Roasting can be done in an oven or grill and results in exceptionally tender foods. The most common types of roasted foods include meats, poultry, fish and vegetables such as peppers, tomatoes and potatoes. For example: roasted baby potatoes, fire roasted red peppers, roast rosemary chicken.

Broiling uses direct, very hot heat from the top of the oven. Fat on meats or in marinades ignites (lights on fire) at this temperature, so you should stick with lean meats, poultry, and fish. This method cooks food in a snap and food can burn quickly. A best practice would be to stay within a few feet of the broiler and check every thirty seconds until you are practiced in broiling. Broiled vegetables and fruits have natural sugars that can develop a caramelized glaze under the broiler that is both crunchy and sweet. Delicious!

The best broiling is done in a standard oven, but a toaster oven can replicate the method if you are patient. The toaster oven doesn't have enough power to generate the intense heat for a true broil, so you end up with a half baked/half broiled meat. Just be sure that it is cooked through to the center. Always pre-heat the oven to achieve a scrumptious meal.

What is preheating an oven?

Put food in a cold oven and your recipe may not turn out quite as planned. Preheat your oven to the desired temperature before baking for an evenly cooked meal.

1. Open the oven and check to see that it is empty and remove anything lurking in there.

2. Move the shelves (before it gets hot) to what the recipe recommends. If it doesn't say, put a shelf in the center of the oven to cook on.

3. Turn or set the temperature to the recipe's stated temperature and setting (usually bake or broil).

4. Wait until the oven reaches this temperature. How do you know? The light will go off (that went on when you turned the oven on), or a digital reading will tell you what temperature it is at. In a toaster oven, wait 10 to 15 minutes if there is no preheat setting.

5. You can prepare your food while the oven is heating. If you wait or forget to heat the oven, nothing much will happen unless you are baking breads, muffins, brownies, pizza crusts, etc. that need to go into a hot oven to rise. You will get a better tasting food if you preheat the oven – it's a good idea!

Grilling is similar to broiling, in that it uses direct heat.
You may know this as barbeque, tailgating, or weenies around the camp fire. There are many types of grills including gas, charcoal, wood-burning and flat-top. The sear is the most important part of grilling. This occurs when you place meat on a very hot heat source. A crust of sorts forms on the outside, holding the natural juices in the meat to get... juicy, not dry. The key is to leave the meat in one place long enough that it gets seared, and then flip it over to sear the other side. Cook until done in the center.

Searing is a technique used to brown the outside of

food. Food can also be seared in a pan or skillet that has been preheated to a high temperature. Think pan-fried steak or fish. Foods that are seared properly will have a crunchy outer crust and tender center. Searing the outside of a beef roast before oven roasting will keep the flavor and juices inside.

Braising involves cooking meats or vegetables in low,

moist heat for a long period of time. Typically, braised foods are seared first, and then transferred to a roasting pan. Braising food creates tender meats and soft vegetables – serious comfort food! Examples would be: pot roast, pork roast for pulled pork, or chicken in wine sauce.

Steaming is cooking method which uses a small

amount of water to quickly cook foods. Vegetables are placed in the basket, which is than placed inside a pot with a lid. A steamer basket comes with many rice cookers so that you can steam vegetables at the same time as cook rice. You can "steam" fresh vegetables in a microwave by rinsing them and leaving a lot of the water on them. Place in a microwave bowl and cover loosely.

Sautéing is a quick-cook method where food is

prepared in a small amount of butter, oil, or water. Literally, it means "to jump." High heat and quick movements to keep the food from staying in one place too long characterize this technique. This is what theatrical chefs are doing when they toss food in a pan for an audience. It's not just for show; it saves time in a busy kitchen.

Meats, vegetables and fruits can be sautéed in a pot, pan or skillet. Preheat the skillet or pan on high before adding the food. The oil is added and the food is tossed around or rapidly stirred or shaken. This method is quick and results in crisp vegetables and meats with a golden crust. Stir-frying is a cousin of the sauté technique.

Boiling is a method of cooking with liquid at high heats.

Common meals would be pastas, soups, stews, or poached meats and fish. Boiling is the action liquids make when they reach 120° degrees F. It is characterized by bubbles of air escaping from the bottom of the pan to the top. Pasta put into hot boiling water will keep its form and structure better than if cooked in simmering water.

Simmering is a cooking technique in which foods are cooked in hot liquids kept at or just barely below the boiling point of water. You would simmer a soup or stew to develop and meld flavors. Poaching fish in aromatic liquid is done at a simmer. After a boil is reached, you turn down the heat on the pan or pot until fine bubbles are released. Many recipes in this and other cookbooks will instruct you to turn the food item down to a simmer, or simmer for say 10-15 minutes. This allows all the foods to continue cooking and release flavor into the dish.

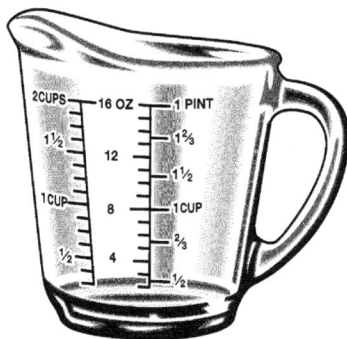

Cooking Measurements

Recipes are often written in an abbreviated style, which can be confusing if you haven't a clue what they mean. This table will help.

Dash	less than 1/8 teaspoon
Tsp., tsp, teas., or t.	teaspoon
Tbsp., tbsp, or T.	tablespoon
C. or c.	one cup
Pt.	one pint (2 cups)
Qt.	one quart (4 cups)
Gal.	one gallon (4 quarts)
Oz. or oz.	one ounce (2 Tablespoons)
Lb. or lb.	one pound (16 ounces)
Pkg.	package
Cont.	container
Min.	minute
Hr.	hour
Deg. or °	degree

Just as important as knowing *what* to measure is *how* to measure. When you use measuring spoons or cups, the object is to get a level measure. If what you're measuring is dry, scoop up extra (called a *well rounded* teaspoon or cup) with the correct measure and **level** off the cup or spoon with the flat side of a knife. If you are measuring liquids, you will almost always *not* get the right amount if you bring it up to eye level. Leave the liquid measure on the counter and bend down to see if the liquid line is at the same level as the marking on the measure.

Most recipes are written for 4 to 6 servings. In this book you will find smaller measurements listed than the normal teaspoon since we are scaling these recipes for one person. Usually, the smallest spoon on a measuring set is ¼ teaspoon. If 1/8 teaspoon is listed, it means fill the ¼ teaspoon half full. This can also be called a "dash."

Food Preparation Terminology

There are many ways to prepare food for cooking. How you cut it can make a difference in the outcome, so it's nice to know what these most common terms mean.

- Slice - To cut food horizontally or vertically into slices.
- Chop - To cut food into irregular pieces or chunks, usually ½" or less in size (or the size of a dime).
- Dice - To cut food into small cubes about ¼" in size (or the size of a pencil top). Commonly used when preparing soups, stews and casseroles.
- Mince - To cut food into tiny pieces. Think garlic or parsley.
- Julienne - To cut into long, thin strips. Nice for stir fry or meats on salads.
- Grate - Food is shredded into fine pieces by rubbing it against a food grater or other rough surface.
- Beat - To make the consistency of food smooth. Food can be beaten with a spoon, fork, whisk, or electric mixer.
- Mix - To combine two or more ingredients together.
- Combine - To mix two or more ingredients together.

Safe knife usage begins with the right knife for the purpose. A paring knife, utility slicing knife and small chef's knife will get you through most of your beginning cooking challenges. They should be sharp and kept in a container for your safety as well as keeping the edges sharp. A plastic pencil case works great for this purpose.

For safe food preparation with a knife, there is the obvious rule of cutting AWAY from your body or hands. Besides that, the single most important thing to remember is to get the knife started cutting into the food before applying pressure to the cutting motion. Many foods like tomatoes and onions have a slippery surface that will try to slide out from under your knife if you're not paying attention. Make sure your knife cuts into the outer skin, and then make your cut. One less trip to the infirmary will be good for your grades!

Reading a Recipe

1.

Read your list of ingredients. Make sure you have all the items before you start following the recipe. You don't want to get half way through the recipe and find you are missing a key ingredient.

2.

Finish reading the whole recipe so that you are aware of all the steps involved.

3.

Make sure you understand the measuring terms. Check that your measuring tools match the recipe and that you understand the measurements.

4.

Pre-heat your oven to the required temperature if you are cooking the food in the oven. This allows you to prepare the recipe while the oven warms up.

5.

Place all the ingredients on the counter in your reach. Get all your measuring cups and measuring spoons ready. Some recipe steps must be performed quickly so you want everything in easy reach. Most recipes list the ingredients in the order of use. If the ingredient needs to be chopped or prepared, you should do this first before the actual combining or cooking.

6.

Follow the steps listed in the recipe paying attention to what each step should look like or the time required.

7.

Mix ingredients together according to recipe directions. Sometimes ingredients need to be mixed together before they can be added to the recipe.

Reading a Recipe, continued

8.

Heat or cook the recipe according to the directions. Make sure your oven is set at the correct temperature or you are cooking at the specified temperature on the stove.

9.

Check the food often while it is cooking. All ovens, microwaves, and appliances heat differently. You may need more or less cooking time than the recipe suggests.

10.

Most recipes are now written without salt and pepper listed, so season to taste with salt and pepper or your own favorite seasonings.

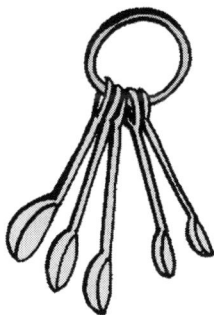

Common Cooking Terms

If you are instructed to... *"Drain the water. "*
This usually refers to draining pasta. The instruction assumes you know to put a colander or sieve in a sink or container that can hold all of the liquid in the pot you are trying to strain. The point is to safely drain all the liquid without burning yourself. You should also keep the food sanitary by not pouring it into a sink and scooping it out. (And yes, I know of someone doing this for real!)

If you are instructed to... *"Cook the pasta until tender. "*
Pasta is tender means that it can easily be pierced with a fork. Traditional tests for wheat based pasta don't always apply to brown rice, corn or quinoa pastas. Stirring gluten free pasta should be a gentle affair, and cook it slightly underdone as the pasta tends to keep absorbing water. Personal note: My first pot of pasta was a broken mess, so experience tells me that the less stirring the better.

If you are instructed to... *"Stir occasionally. "*
Stir once in a while to keep the food from sticking to the bottom of the pan or to itself. *Stirring frequently* means to watch the pot and stir almost constantly. Good stirring is not an act of whirlpool aggression. Instead, gently scrape the spoon around the bottom of the pot and keep the contents moving.

If you are instructed to... *"Heat the oil in a skillet. "*
Heating the oil means to place it in a skillet, turn on the heat to medium, and leaving the oil on the heat for 1-2 minutes, until you can feel the warmth when you hold your hand 3-4 inches above the pan.

If you are instructed to... *"Cook on medium heat. "*
Usually this refers to stovetop cooking and how hot you should turn the dial to. Medium heat is half way on your dial. If numbered (often 1 to 8), that means 4 on a scale of 8. Medium high heat would be 6, and low heat would be about 2. Keep warm would be the lowest setting or 1. Remember, you can always turn the heat up, but overcooking food is permanent!

If you are instructed to..."*Brown the ground beef*"
This works for ground turkey and chicken too. Browning the
ground beef means to cook just until the pink or red color
disappears. Stir with a fork or non-stick spoon so the larger
piece of ground beef breaks up as it cooks. You should have
small uniform pieces when done. This does NOT mean to cook
until the meat turns the color of burnt toast.

If you are instructed to... "*Drain the fat.*"
Usually from the aforementioned ground meat, this means to
safely pour off the hot fat in the pan into a container that will
not melt. DO NOT pour fat into the drain. DO NOT pour hot fat
into anything that has had water or a liquid in it as it will
splatter. It's not fun to be showered with hot grease, so listen up.
Pour hot fat into a metal container (think clean and empty
aluminum can), and allow the fat to cool to room temperature.
Scoop it out into your garbage. Recycle the can.

**If you are instructed to... "*Cook onions/vegetables
until translucent or soft.*"**
Cooking onions until translucent means the color of the onions
changes from pure white to a softer, more transparent, white.
Cooking vegetables until they *"start to soften"* means that they
are no longer crisp and firm, but start to be flexible and soft.

**If you are instructed to... "*Cook vegetables until
tender.*"**
Means that when you poke or pierce them with a fork, the tines
of the fork slide easily into the flesh, with little resistance. If you
like crisp vegetables go with the brightness of the color. Most
vegetables get a vibrant color just before they become "tender."
It's your choice – tender or crisp.

If you are instructed to... "*Grease the pan.*"
Usually for baked goods or casseroles. Grease pans by rubbing
them with a bit of gluten free shortening, oil, margarine or
butter, _or_ spraying with gluten free nonstick cooking spray. The
shortening should be a very thin, even coating over every inside
surface - so the pan is shiny. No shortening should be visible.

Appliances for the College Dorm

Every college has a different set of rules about what appliances are allowed in dorm rooms. There are many reasons for this, but safety usually outranks any others. Dorms built before a decade ago are not set up for the electrical demand that modern technology puts on college buildings. While constant improvements are made on each campus for the demands and safety of the residents, appliances may not be allowed because of the electrical draw. Personal responsibility is also an issue.

In a worst case scenario, you might just be allowed a mini refrigerator in the room. Another college may allow all sorts of appliances with permission. There is a wide discrepancy among colleges on this point. One of the first questions you should ask the university admissions/housing department is whether there is an "allowable appliance list." Also ask if there are any exceptions for hidden disabilities like food allergy/intolerance. In many contemporary dorms, there will be a shared kitchenette area for cooking. While this may be acceptable, the cross contamination issues may not be. Ask to see the cooking areas (and on more than one floor of the dorm) so that you can really evaluate the environment.

Real estate in a dorm room is valuable. Every thing that goes in it (including an extra room mate sometimes) has to have a small footprint. Plan for this and you will be happy in your new home. Let's look at some advantages and disadvantages of dorm size appliances:

Mini Refrigerators. Each college or university has a list of acceptable makes and models. It's a good idea to wait to buy or rent until you know absolutely which models are allowed. The college will have a policy on this or rental information. A mini refrigerator has mini space. There is not a lot of room in a small refrigerator for food (after condiments and soda) so canned or aseptic packaged groceries may be the best bet for stocking the dorm pantry.

Microwaves. Usually only a very low wattage microwave is allowed – if at all. You may be able to use one you have at home but you will need to know the college policy. A small microwave is really all that is needed anyway and may fit the space better than a high powered version.

Toaster Oven. If these are allowed, it will have to be a small one. The electrical draw will be a limiting factor in choosing an approved model. If the student is handy with baking from gluten free mixes, a toaster oven can come in handy over a regular toaster because it can broil tostadas or bake pizza crusts. If allowed, it would be a good addition.

Rice Cooker. If limited for space, this appliance is the one item I would recommend in addition to a refrigerator. A rice cooker can make a wide variety of foods with a very small electrical usage and safe operation – it shuts itself off. Although some colleges don't even allow a hot pot, you may be able to negotiate for this appliance. You can reheat, cook, make breakfast, create casseroles and stews, and even make grilled cheese in this appliance. A 3-6 cup rice cooker is perfect for one person. It makes one to four portions perfectly. The larger capacity cookers tend to dry out smaller portion sizes for one or two people.

A big box store (think red circle) sells a red model marked 6 cup capacity which is a 3 cup rice cooker. Rice cookers are sold by the number of cups of rice, 3 in this case, which is a 6 cup capacity. (Rice doubles in size when cooked.) This is confusing but once you see a 3 cup size model, you will be able to recognize the size. These cost under $20.00 at discount stores. Consider buying one with a non-stick lining for easy clean up, and with a steamer basket included (doubles as a colander).

Electric Skillet. This is similar to a rice cooker in capabilities, but doesn't heat larger quantities of liquids well because of the short sides (think boiling water for pasta). However, the skillet will make pancakes or grilled cheese sandwiches, so it may be a trade off. Smaller size 12" skillets are now available.

Electric Wok. Real stir-frying requires more heat than an electric model can usually muster. But, if you live on stir fried veggies and Asian foods, this would work for heating or cooking most foods including boiling water for pasta or noodles.

Toaster. If the student lives on gluten free bread, this is worth asking for a special allowance to have one of these on the basis of cross contamination alone.

Blender. Unless you live on smoothies or protein shakes, this will just take up space. The smaller bullet size blenders can come in handy for smoothies, chopping vegetables, etc. depending on the needs of the student.

Clamshell or Panini Grill. Grilling raw meats is probably beyond what will be considered safe in a dorm room, so this will usually not be on the approved list. They are great for the college apartment if you have the room.

Waffle Iron. A waffle iron and a simple to use pancake mix could be just the thing for a waffle lover. It is very economical to make your own waffles and freeze a few for quick meals.

Hot Pot. You can heat water and soup in this appliance, but not a whole lot more. For the same size, you could have a rice cooker that does so much more.

Please keep in mind that these appliances may not be on the college's allowed model list. You may ask for an exception because of dietary requirements, or cross contamination issues with gluten. Negotiation skills will help you in this process. If an appliance is against fire code there will be no recourse, and shouldn't be. Follow the safety rules of your particular college – they are there for a reason!

Why a Rice Cooker ?

A rice cooker is a very unique appliance often overlooked in most American kitchens. However, it does much more than just cooking perfect rice. First, it is safe because it turns itself to a *keep warm setting* when it gets close to done. Have you ever heard of a stove doing that? Secondly, it boils water which means you can cook pasta, or reheat soups, or prepare anything you can cook in a saucepan. You can even steam other foods in the steamer basket while the bottom is cooking something else. Below are some tips about this appliance.

◆ Rice cookers are classified by the type of appliance they are – basic, electronic, or micom (microcomputer). The basic model with a cook and keep warm setting is all you need for student cooking.

◆ Rice cookers are sold by the amount of uncooked rice they can typically cook. A rice cooker that says its *capacity is **6 cups cooked rice*** would be considered a ***3 cup machine***.

◆ A small rice cooker would be a 3 to 4 cup machine and is suitable for 1-3 people. Available for under $20 at most big box stores, it fits the budget nicely!

◆ Rice, grains, or many other foods may be cooked in any version of a rice cooker.

◆ A rice cooker is very energy efficient and the steamer basket may be used for multiple purposes (steaming, reheating) while cooking rice or grains. You can steam vegetables and cook rice at the same time.

◆ The "keep warm" function of the rice cooker will keep your foods warm until you turn it off (or it is programmed to turn off). Always remove the electric cord from the outlet to completely turn off your rice cooker.

◆ Can help reduce **cross contamination issues** in a multi person residence *if used only for gluten free cooking*.

How a Rice Cooker Works

As if by magic, the rice cooker senses when the rice is done. It's not really magic – it's done by a thermostat – that mimics the best intentions of the busy cook to watch what's cooking on the stove.

How is it that the rice cooker "knows" when to switch off or to warm automatically? The rice cooker works by a thermal sensing device that is activated when the temperature changes in the cooking pan. When rice and liquid is placed into the inner cooking pan and then placed into the cooking chamber, the weight of the cooking ingredients will depress the thermal sensor.

When the rice cooker is plugged in and turned on to the cook setting, the heating plate starts to bring the ingredients to a boil. Since water boils at 212° F. and will not go higher, the rice cooker will continue to cook only until there is no water left. Once the ingredients have absorbed all the liquid, the temperature begins to rise in the cooking chamber. The thermal sensor will switch the cooker to the "keep warm" setting when the temperature rises above 212° F. So very simple and efficient!

Most basic rice cookers have two settings – a "keep warm" setting and a "cook" setting. When cooking a dense food like breakfast strata or ground meat, the cooker may flip to the keep warm setting during cooking. *Wait for a couple of minutes for the temperature to drop in the cooking well* and then flip the switch to cook again for more direct heat. The keep warm setting on most cookers is about 180° degrees F. (well above the 165° degrees F. recommended for safety). It will continue to cook, just *slowly*.

*C*ooking Tip...
If you are cooking rice or grains, the cooker will turn to warm when the liquid has evaporated. If you are using it to cook more solid foods, you will need to *manually move the switch* between high and keep warm depending on how much heat the food needs that you are cooking.

Things You Can Make in a Rice Cooker

No, this is not an ad to sell rice cookers, but the truth is that it is an excellent appliance for small meal cooking. It is wonderfully versatile for more than cooking rice, and it is one of the safest appliances around. Your culinary imagination is the only limit on what you foods you can prepare in this appliance. For size and portability, it can't be beat.

Scrambled Eggs.

♦ **Crack** 2-3 eggs into a bowl and add a splash of milk (or alternative milk). Season with salt and pepper. Beat well with a fork. Pour into the rice cooker and turn on to high setting. Use a heat resistant spatula to move the eggs around as they cook. Note: if using a rice cooker that is not non-stick coated, you should add a small amount of oil before adding the eggs.

Heat frozen waffles.

♦ **Butter** the waffle on both sides lightly with margarine or butter. Put in rice cooker and turn on to high setting. Flip over when one side is browned, cook on other side until brown. Makes a crispy, crunchy waffle to top with syrup or applesauce.

Quick soups. *Heat from a can or make your own.*

♦ **Quick** tomato soup – Combine one cup of pasta cooking sauce with ½ c. milk or milk substitute. Heat until bubbly.
♦ **Quick** chicken noodle – Heat one cup chicken broth until boiling. Add broken up rice noodle sticks and cook for 5 minutes. Spice it up with soy sauce or tamari, leftover meats or vegetables.

Hot breakfast cereal

♦ Combine the hot cereal with the recommended amount of water or apple juice. The cereal may boil over if covered tightly, put the cover on but leave it ajar. Turn on the rice cooker to high heat setting, stirring occasionally until thick and creamy. Add dried fruit, cinnamon or applesauce to spice up your morning.

Cook pasta and rice noodles.

♦ For Pasta: Fill rice cooker half full with water – turn on
  and cover. Add ½ c. to 1 c. rice pasta when the water has
  started to boil. Cook until mostly done, about 8 minutes.
  Cover and turn the cooker to warm for 5 minutes. Drain.
  Add sauce and heat, or use the cooked pasta for salad or as
  an ingredient in another recipe.

♦ For Rice Noodles: Fill rice cooker half full with water –
  turn on and cover. Drop rice noodles into boiling water in
  the rice cooker and turn to warm after 2 minutes, cover. In
  8 minutes, you will have perfect rice noodles. Drain and
  use with oriental foods or to make cold sesame noodles.

Cooking Tip...
You can drain pasta or noodles through the steamer basket
that comes with a rice cooker – it makes a great colander!

Sauté cooked fajita meat and vegetables.

♦ Put 1 teaspoon of oil in the rice cooker with sliced onions
  and peppers (about ½ cup). Turn on to high heat and stir
  as the food cooks. When the peppers start to soften, add
  cooked meats or protein cut in strips – beef, chicken, or
  tofu – and add fajita or Mexican seasoning. Continue to
  cook until hot. Eat as is or fill a gluten free wrap.

Stir Fry meats & vegetables.

♦ Put 1 teaspoon of oil in the rice cooker with raw vegetables
  and cooked meat or tofu. Turn on and stir as the food
  heats. Finish with soy sauce or tamari, a drizzle of sesame
  oil, or oriental seasoning.

Things You Can Make in a Rice Cooker~ Continued

Cook a hamburger or turkey burger.

♦ Form the raw ground meat into a patty that is ½" thick or less. Put into the rice cooker and turn on high heat. As the edges begin to cook, turn over and cook the other side. Don't forget your favorite seasoning or sauce. The best way to make sure the burger is done is to test with a food thermometer to 165° F.

Grill a chicken breast.

♦ Put one teaspoon of cooking oil in the rice cooker with the boneless chicken breast. Turn on high heat. Turn over when one side is browned. Cover in between. Add 2 Tbsp. of water to the cooker and cover – cook for 5-8 minutes more. To test if done, use a meat thermometer to read 165° F. when inserted horizontally into the center of the chicken breast.

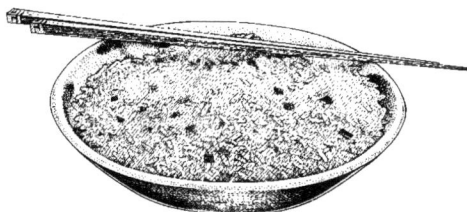

Suggested Kitchen Equipment

Getting by with the bare minimum in kitchen utensils can become an art form in any tight space, but especially in cramped college living spaces. This is a basic suggestion list for general food preparation needs, as well as the recipes in this book. The good news is that most of these items can be purchased at a dollar or discount store. In fact, that would be encouraged since personal items are easily lost or misplaced in a group living setting.

Small cutting board
Silicone hot pads (2)
Stirring spoons, plastic
High heat spatula
Sandwich spreader
Non-stick pancake turner
Plastic soup ladle
Plastic large serving spoon
Non-stick potato masher
Paring knife
Serrated slicing knife, 4-6"
Chef's knife, 6"
Microwave safe pie plate
Microwave safe clear 2 cup measure
Microwave safe 2 quart container w/ lid

Vegetable peeler
Can opener
Collapsible colander
Collapsible storage bowls
Food thermometer
Refrigerator thermometer
Storage bags
Plastic wrap
Wax paper for microwaving
Set of dry measuring cups
Set of measuring spoons
Plate and cereal bowls

Sanitation Items:

Anti-bacterial wipes/spray
Hand Sanitizer
Disposable towels

Dish detergent
Dish scrubber
Vegetable brush

Foods Used in the Recipes

The dorm or college apartment kitchen is usually very limited in refrigeration space, cooking utensils, and storage space. This also limits the amounts of gluten free ingredients the dorm cook can have in their pantry. The recipes in this book were designed with just a few special ingredients.

Special gluten free foods you may need for some of the recipes:

- ♦ Gluten free flour mix
- ♦ Gluten free pancake mix
- ♦ All purpose gluten free baking mix

Breads
- ♦ Gluten free rice or teff wraps
- ♦ Corn tostadas
- ♦ Gluten free bread

Thickeners:
- ♦ Cornstarch, potato starch, or arrowroot

Baking Ingredients:
- ♦ Baking powder
- ♦ Baking soda
- ♦ Vanilla
- ♦ Dry vanilla powder for select recipes

A few of the recipes use Xanthan gum. While this is an expensive initial purchase, a bag will probably last one person six months to a year. You need very little to make a big difference in baked goods. Keep it in a dry, sealed container. Always mix the Xanthan with the dry ingredients before adding liquids.

Every effort was made to design the recipes with common gluten free ingredients that are available on or near college campuses. Experienced gluten free cooks can always elaborate on the basic recipes. The *beginning cook* should be able to complete any recipe in this book for a quality, satisfying meal.

Suggested Seasonings

The difference between good cooking and great cooking is in the seasoning. Whole spices are generally considered safe for gluten free cooking. When spices get mixed together commercially, the level of contamination can increase from manufacturing binders or additives used to stabilize the spices. For this reason, unless a manufacturer specifically confirms that their seasoning mixes are gluten free, you should steer clear until you can verify the gluten free status.

The good news is that spice and seasoning mixes are very easy to make. Your home-crafted spice blends can be customized to exclude herbs you may be sensitive to. They will also cost substantially less if you make them, rather than a food manufacturer. The chapter titled Condiments and Seasonings has several different spice mixes you can use to flavor food for great taste. Herb and spice blends are fabulous Gifts from Home in a care package.

Try to avoid buying large amounts of herbs or spices as they taste better when fresh. Most seasonings should be used within 6 months. You may want to raid your parents seasoning stash when at home, using small sealable plastic bags to take just a small amount with you to college. Otherwise, share (the cost too!) among other students you know who like to cook. You can purchase herbs and spices in small quantities from many health food stores, but you must be certain that there are no cross contamination issues with their products. In general, it is best to stay away from bulk buying on the gluten free diet.

S hopping Tip:
The recipes in this book were created using the following blends and spices. These recommendations are just suggestions. You can judge for yourself which seasonings will be most important for your cooking style and taste.

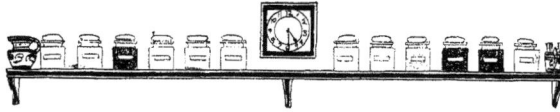

Basic spices for a college spice rack:

Basil
Oregano
Garlic powder
Onion powder
Dehydrated onion flakes
Salt
Pepper
Cinnamon
Red pepper flakes
Dill
Chili powder
Cumin
Sage
Dry mustard (for macaroni and cheese)

Seasoning blends for convenience:

All purpose seasoning
Italian seasoning or pizza seasoning
Taco or Mexican Seasoning

International cooking sauces and spices:

Thai Chili Sauce
Green curry paste
Red curry paste
Curry Powder
Toasted Sesame Oil
Wheat free tamari, or soy sauce

Other sauces and condiments:

Gluten free bouillon cubes or powder
or stock in small aseptic packages
Hot pepper sauce
Worcestershire sauce
Ketchup
Prepared mustard, Dijon mustard

Grocery Shopping at College

Hey, you're a solo shopper! You'll soon find that shopping for one is very frustrating. Most meats and some produce are packaged for small families. When items are packaged singly the price of the item often skyrockets - from added labor and costly individual packaging. However, you should think of this as a challenge that you <u>will</u> immediately overcome. The gluten free college student is just a wiser shopper!

Shopping On Campus.

Let's take a moment and discuss the meaning of "convenience" as in **Convenience Stores**. Most C-stores are higher in price when compared to a grocery store. A few of the reasons are that they don't buy in grocery store volume; they don't have a lot of shelf space to inventory products; and their delivery charges are higher for small shipments. Therefore, it costs more—a lot more!

On the other hand, the store is *on campus,* and usually within walking distance. In other words – *very convenient.* Depending on the school, you may be able to use your foodservice dollars at the convenience stores. This is how colleges are able to provide these stores on campus for use of the students. It costs more, but you don't have to drive to get what you want.

To make the best use of your convenience store, ask them to stock items you will use. The people who run the stores like to get products that people will buy, so be specific with brand and size. Also let them know how much you will pay for it. It is terrible to stock a product and have no one buy it because of the price. This discourages the food service management from stocking any item that's slightly unusual.

Enlist the aid of the campus dietician to help identify gluten free products for the on campus store managers. There may not be a wide variety of gluten free products available through the store suppliers, but this will change as the demand increases.

In the meantime, ask that the dining service offer pre-cut or prepared vegetables, salads, or sliced meats that are gluten free in the convenience stores. Many traditional cafeterias are also offering grocery items that can be purchased when you are there for a meal.

Shopping Off Campus.

Supermarkets.

Rarely will there be a market close to a campus with a large selection of gluten free foods. Real estate is either too dear in a city, or if the college town is in the country, the town may not be large enough to justify an expansive gluten free section. You may have to make a weekly or bi-weekly trip to a store that carries your favorite items.

If most of your meals come from the dining options on campus, you will just want to stock up on things that may not be offered at the foodservice. Specifically, pasta that you like, favorite breads and wraps, nutritious grains like brown rice and quinoa, and gluten free sauces or dressings. It is a good idea to make a running list of grocery store items on your computer that you check off when you need them. Just print out the list so you don't forget anything on a once-in-a-while shopping trip.

Shopping for one person at the grocery store:

This may be the single most difficult challenge of eating gluten free at college – knowing where and how to buy smaller quantities of food than is normally packaged and sold in grocery stores. Here are some suggestions...

♦ At a grocery store, use the staffed deli and butcher sections for small portions. If you only want ¼ pound of ground meat this is the place to go. Order your meat items in ¼ pound increments. Think of a quarter pound hamburger and you will get the idea of how many "quarter pounds" of raw meat you want. You can also get just one pork chop or one chicken breast. Ignore any strange looks from the counter person and ask for what you want. They should also be able to tell or show you an ingredient label from meat items that have been marinated or injected with broth. Making friends with a butcher can be one of the best things you can do on a gluten free diet. As they get to know you, they will alert you to other gluten free items you may like.

♦ A typical overstuffed sandwich contains about 2 ½ to 3 oz. of cooked sandwich meat. If you order ½ pound of deli meat (or 8 oz.), you will have about 3 portions of meat. Most deli departments will cut meat down to ¼ pound but not below that. Ask nice and explain your situation – most people will like to help.

♦ The salad bar. You don't have to make *just salad* from the salad bar! This is where you can find an assortment of vegetables all precut and in the quantity that you need. A whole head of broccoli may be too much for one person, but you can get a cup of already cut broccoli from the salad bar. This is an excellent place to get oriental vegetables for stir-fry. Think sliced mushrooms, baby corn, water chestnuts, green and red peppers, broccoli, or onions. You can get several meals of vegetables in one container all ready to go into the pan. Be wary of cross contamination issues. This may not be an option for everyone.

♦ The grab n' go area of the produce section. Many stores now carry cut onions, peppers, celery, etc in the convenience section. Be aware that you pay for them to pre-cut these items, so if you are on a strict budget, it is best to learn how to cut up an onion or pepper on your own. They are less likely to have cross contamination than a salad bar but that only depends on how they are prepared in the kitchen. Ask the store manager for more information.

Health Food Stores. It is very possible that there
will be a health food store near a major university, or in most towns. This is a great place to stock up on alternative milks, cheeses, spices, rice, grains, stock, tamari sauce, etc. You may find these stores more responsive to ordering special items for you. They will likely have other customers who also may want the items.

Oriental Markets. The plus side to an oriental

grocery is that you can buy rice sticks (noodles) of all sizes, coconut milk, a wide variety of rice, and rice flours at one half to one quarter the price of a product made in a gluten free facility in the U. S.

But, and this is a BIG BUT, while lower cost sounds great, there is no guarantee that the imported items have not been cross contaminated by wheat in production. If you are very sensitive to gluten, it is a poor idea to purchase products made in a non-gluten free facility whatever the country of origin. It is up to you to decide if these products are for you.

Support Groups. A new trend is local support groups

that "adopt" a college student and help them with acquiring items they need. Contact the local celiac support group before you go to get the locations of stores and restaurants in your spending range.

Care Packages from Home. One of the best

ways parents can support their college student is with a gluten free goodie bag once in a while. Don't forget the option to get an online order from gluten free sites sent directly to your student at school.

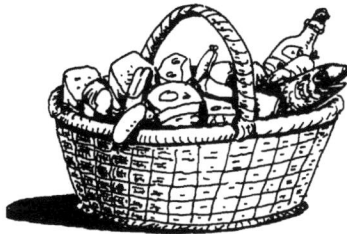

Safe Food Handling

Preparing food safely is just as important as the taste of the food. The news is full of reports on bacterial infections or "food poisoning" outbreaks. So how do you keep yourself free of food related digestive troubles? Here are some very basic guidelines to help you understand the issues:

Wash Your Hands. Before, during, and after food
preparation. This is the best way to prevent unwanted bacteria from traveling from one food to another. We all know about cross contamination with gluten, and the same rules apply for cross contamination with illness-causing bacteria on food. When working with raw meats or unwashed fruits and vegetables, always clean the preparation areas, utensils and your hands in hot soapy water before using them for something else. Sanitize surfaces with disinfectant wipes or sprays and do not re-use towels that have come into contact with raw meats.

Keep Food Cold. Room temperature is the danger
zone for bacteria to grow and spoil food (from 40°F. to 140°F.). Leaving food out on the counter or in a backpack for over 2 hours allows the bacteria process to accelerate. Plan ahead and pack food in a thermal bag if you will not be able to eat it within 2 hours of it being out of the refrigerator. This also applies to any "grab and go" foods from food service. Carry a lightweight, collapsible thermal bag in your knapsack for food.

Potentially Dangerous Foods. Yep, that's
right. That's what they call them at Food Safety Certifications. These are foods that carry an extra risk for bacterial growth: raw meats, dairy products, dry foods that have been cooked (rice, pasta, potatoes, onions, etc), and unwashed fruits or vegetables to name a few. Always refrigerate these items immediately and take care to wash all produce before eating.

Wash Food Well. Any produce grown in soil may
carry unwanted bacteria. Hold foods under running water

and use a food brush to lightly scrub the surface of whole fruits or vegetables. Wash lettuce by the leaf and drain well. Running water, not soaking, will wash away the visible dirt, and the invisible bacteria.

Wash Your Hands Often. When cooking raw
meats, there should be a hand sink nearby. You will need to wash your hands for 15 seconds with soap before and after working with raw meat, poultry or fish. If a hand washing facility is not nearby, then you should not work with raw meats – use canned or pre-cooked instead. A dorm room may not be a place to cook raw meats, but the kitchenette or apartment kitchen may be appropriate.

Sanitize Surfaces. When working with potentially
hazardous foods, you must be careful to sanitize the work area, the utensils and knives, cutting boards, and not re-use towels. You can sanitize these items by washing in hot, soapy water and allowing them to air dry on a clean surface; run through a dishwasher if available; or use kitchen wipes treated with anti-bacterial chemicals *for surfaces*. Do not spray dishes or eating utensils with anti-bacterial spray – use hot soapy water to clean up anything you eat on or with.

Cook It Through. There are safe temperatures for
every kind of food. If there is a *mixture of foods* like a casserole, stew or ground meat, the temperature of the food should reach 165° Fahrenheit in the center of the food. This is the temperature where most bacteria are killed. Bacteria hang out on the surface of food, so when you cook a steak to 130° F. in the center for medium rare, you remove the danger on the outside because the temperature reaches over 165°F. *on the surface.* When you have ground meat, all the surfaces are mixed together and need to all reach 165°F. That is why burgers are now all cooked well done in most restaurants.

How to tell when 165°F. is reached? The only accurate way is to use a simple food thermometer. The stem end is placed in the middle of the cooked product and the temperature is allowed to register. What is the center of a hamburger? You put the thermometer in the side of the patty (horizontal) until the thermometer reaches the center. This works for a chicken breast too. The old test of "seeing the juices run clear" is now considered un-safe. Using a simple thermometer is the best food safety precaution.

Cool It Down. Once foods are mixed together, they need to be cooled down quickly. Store leftovers in containers that are more wide than deep. Allow the food to cool to room temperature, cover and refrigerate. Never put really hot things in your refrigerator – it will make the temperature in the refrigerator warm up and put all the food at risk. Leftover food in small amounts should be refrigerated within 1/2 hour.

Refrigerator Temperature. Keeping food cold is the key. What is cold? It should register between 36° - 39° F. It is a good practice to keep a refrigerator thermometer in your fridge so you can check occasionally. If your refrigeration stops working, all the food in it is not safe if the temperature rises above 40°F. for more than a short period of time.

Safe Food Storage Times. Expiration dates are important to read. As a rule, you should cook or freeze raw meat within one to two days. Leftovers should be eaten or discarded within one or two days as well. Reheat foods to 165°F. in the center.

Wash the Dishes and Take The Garbage Out. Clean up is just as important as cooking. Be a friend to yourself and the people you live with and "clean as you go."
For further information, please see the U. S. Food Safety website, www.foodsafety.gov , and especially this brochure *Food Safety Tips for College Students.*

Cross Contamination in Group Settings

Living with other people can be interesting. There is a lot of give and take among roommates at college and after. If you can find a gluten free roommate, you will have eliminated a great deal of concern. If not, here is a list of good practices to discuss with your dorm or apartment mates.

- Even small amounts of gluten can result in continued intestinal damage for people with gluten intolerance so be on constant alert for *wheat crumbs*.

- Devise a labeling system that you and your roommates can agree on and respect. Colored labels or markers may come in handy for this on-going project.

- Can regular food stored in a refrigerator contaminate gluten free food also stored there? Yes, if it is not tightly sealed or packaged. The best policy would be to have at minimum an upper shelf for GF foods, or even a separate dorm size refrigerator just for GF. Wash the refrigerator surfaces often.

- Double dipping is not good. Separate jars of condiments may be necessary because of wheat crumbs, etc. Label the GF ones. Single serve condiment packets may be practical if you are living with many people.

- Separate utensils, kitchen tools, and pans can contain residual gluten. Stick with plastic tools over wood, and stainless steal pans over non-stick coated if you must share. Glass or ceramic baking pans can be scrubbed cleaner than metal.

- A toaster or toaster oven of your very own – well labeled "gluten free foods ONLY."

Cross Contamination ~ Continued

♦ Clean any surface that is used to prepare foods with gluten before using it to prepare GF foods. Remember, gluten proteins must be washed away – you cannot sanitize it away with antibacterial wipes.

♦ Therefore, it follows that separate cutting boards would be a good thing. Or, make your GF foods first on the board, then the gluten containing version second. Wash the board very well before and after use.

♦ The common use microwave should be avoided at all costs, unless there is no other option. It should be wiped down very well before putting gluten free items in it. Add a second layer of protection by covering your foods with plastic or vented covers. Don't let the bottom of the microwave container sit on a surface that you may prepare food on latter - in case there are crumbs sticking to it.

♦ After handling or cleaning up gluten containing foods, wash your hands. Crumbs, flour or barley ingredients can easily pass onto your food.

♦ And speaking of cleaning up, using sponges that have wiped up gluten containing foods on counters will spread more gluten when you use them again. A dish scrubby riddled with gluten foods will not leave your dishes gluten free. A separate scrubby would be a good idea. For wiping up, disposable towels are not environmentally friendly, but may be your only choice in a group living situation to prevent getting sick.

♦ Work with the college or university housing department months before you get to college to find a like-minded roommate. After your first semester, you will likely know more students with gluten intolerance and be able to make a change if needed.

Enjoy a healthy and productive college career!

The Recipes

Gluten Free College Student Cookbook

Sweet and Salty Things

Perfect snack attacks for any time of day

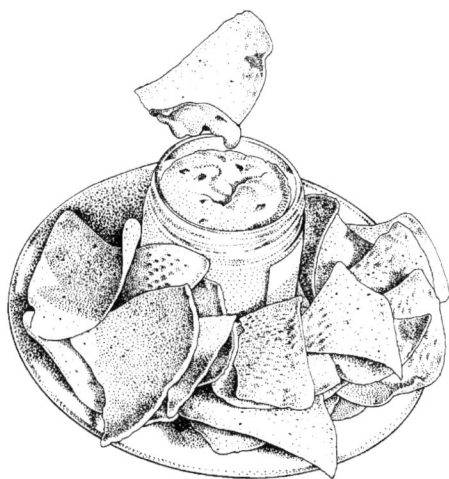

Sweet and salty. Crave one, crave them all. Snacks are the new meal.

The so called "fourth meal" is nothing but a big snack for hungry students at midnight. In fact, midnight is often the middle of the day for many students. So to ease the pain of not having great gluten free snacks available at that time of night (or at all!), here are some selections that will definitely get you through the wee hours until dawn.

Note: Items listed in **bold** in the recipes have a higher incidence of containing gluten – it's a *reminder* to always check the label or directly with the manufacturer.

Pizza Fondue

Dip in bread, crackers, pepper strips, or chips...

Ingredients:
- ♦ 1/2 cup **pizza sauce**
- ♦ 2 oz. meltable **soy cheese** or dairy American cheese
- ♦ 1/2 tsp. oregano
- ♦ 1 oz. **pepperoni**, diced

Rice Cooker or Stovetop Directions:
Combine all ingredients in rice cooker or 1-quart saucepan. Turn cooker on (stovetop medium low heat) and stir often when the mixture starts to bubble. Cheese should melt completely. Makes 2 portions.

Microwave Directions:
Combine all ingredients in a 2-cup microwavable container. Cover loosely and microwave on 70 % power for 5 minutes. Stir and continue cooking on high until cheese is melted. Makes 2 portions.

Nutrition Information...
Calories: 216   Protein: 8 g   Carbs: 9 g   Fat: 15 g

*V*egan Friendly...
Instead of pepperoni add fresh chopped vegetables or slices of sun-dried tomatoes or olives.

*C*reative Cooking...
Add crumbled sausage, onions and peppers, or pesto sauce for extra flavor.
Dip gluten free toasted bread, crackers, tortilla chips/scoops, or pepper strips into the fondue.

Quick Nacho Sauce

*Great over more than nachos –
try it over chicken, rice, or pasta*

Ingredients:

- 2 oz. **soy nacho cheese**, or dairy cheese (American, Monterey Jack, etc.)
- 1/4 cup **rice, soy, almond, or dairy milk**
- 2 Tbsp. green chilies, diced (optional)
- 1/4 tsp. taco seasoning (optional)

Microwave Directions:

Combine all ingredients in a 2 cup microwave safe container. Cook covered and vented on high for 2 minutes. Stir and continue to cook in 15 second intervals until cheese has melted. Allow to cool for 4-5 minutes. Pour over tortilla chips.

Nutrition Information...
Calories: 248   Protein: 6 g   Carbs: 13 g   Fat: 15 g

*C*reative Cooking...
Load 'em up with jalapeno slices, salsa, diced tomatoes, diced fresh peppers, or crumbled cooked bacon.

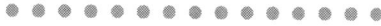

Crispy Corn Tortilla Chips

Hot and crunchy – enjoy with salsa or melt cheese on top

Ingredients:
- ♦ 2 **corn tortillas**
- ♦ cooking oil spray, or vegetable oil
- ♦ 1/2 tsp. **taco seasoning**
- ♦ 1/4 tsp. salt

Microwave Directions:

Lay the tortillas out on a cutting board, lightly spray, brush or mist both sides with oil, then cut each tortilla into six wedges. Place the wedges in a single layer on the microwave oven platter. Microwave on high for 1 1/2 minutes. Turn the tortilla wedges over and microwave for another 1 1/2 minutes.

Continue turning and microwaving at 1 1/2-minute intervals, moving the wedges around if some seem to be browning more than others are, until they are crisp - remember, as they cool, they'll crisp even more. Total microwaving time is likely to be 5-7 minutes. Immediately dust the chips with salt and the taco seasoning.

Oven/Toaster Oven Directions:

Preheat the oven to 450°F. Lay the tortillas out on a cutting board, lightly spray, brush or mist both sides with oil, then cut each tortilla into six wedges. Place the wedges in a single layer on a toaster oven tray. Put in the oven and cook for 5-10 minutes, turning once. Continue to cook until light brown. Immediately dust the chips with salt and the taco seasoning.

Nutrition Information:
Calories: 109   Protein: 3 g   Carbs: 22 g   Fat: 1.5 g

Avocado Mash

May be the ugliest dip ever, but it sure tastes good

Ingredients:
- 1 avocado, seed removed and scooped from skin
- 2 Tbsp. **Ranch salad dressing**, or other creamy dressing
- 1/4 tsp. **hot pepper sauce**, or crushed red pepper

Recipe Directions:
Scoop the avocado out of the skin into a small bowl. Using a fork, mash the avocado until smooth. Add the ranch dressing and hot sauce, and mix well. Use as a dip, spread in wraps or quesadillas, or as a topping for baked potatoes.

Nutrition Information:
Calories: 231   Protein: 2 g   Carbs: 10 g   Fat: 22 g

*V**egan Friendly...***
Use vegan salad dressing instead of dairy based dressing.

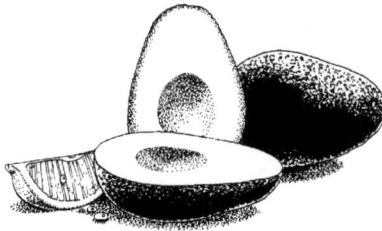

Polenta Nachos

A quick way to turn purchased polenta into a classic snack

Ingredients:

- ♦ 4 slices **polenta** from purchased tube
- ♦ cooking oil spray
- ♦ 1/4 cup **nacho soy cheese**, cubed; or, dairy Monterey jack cheese, shredded
- ♦ 2 Tbsp. salsa
- ♦ 2 Tbsp. jalapeno pepper slices (optional)

Recipe Directions:

Preheat the toaster oven to 400° degrees F. Line a baking sheet with foil.

Cut four 3/8" slices from the polenta log. Lay out on the baking sheet. Lightly spray the polenta on both sides with the cooking spray. Bake for 12-14 minutes, or until the polenta starts to get a crisp crust. Remove from the oven and top each with a spoonful of salsa. Add shredded cheese and jalapeno slices if desired. Put back into the oven on BROIL for 5-10 minutes, or until the cheese is melted.

Nutrition Information:
Calories: 260   Protein: 10 g   Carbs: 35 g   Fat: 8 g

*B*udget Tip...
     Making your own polenta is easy and it can be formed into a log with plastic wrap. Refrigerate and cut as needed.

• • • • • • • • • • • • • •

Southwest Chip Dip

*Great with corn tortilla chips or in a gluten free wrap
with crisp vegetables*

Ingredients:

- ◆ 4 oz. **non-dairy or dairy cream cheese**
- ◆ 1/2 cup **non-dairy or dairy sour cream**
- ◆ 1/2 cup salsa, as hot as you like
- ◆ 1 Tbsp. **taco seasoning mix** (see recipe page 119)

Recipe Directions:

Measure out the cream cheese and let it come to room temperature so it's soft, about a half hour. Mix the sour cream and cream cheese together with a spoon until smooth. Add the salsa and seasoning, stirring well. Chill for 1/2 hour for best flavor. Top with diced tomato, olives, peppers or other favorite taco toppings. Makes 4 servings.

Nutrition Information:
Calories: 193   Protein: 2 g   Carbs: 18 g   Fat: 16 g

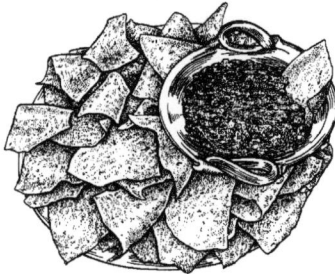

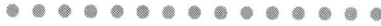

Chili Corn Tortilla Chips

Hot from the oven these chips are perfect with salsa or with melted cheese as nachos

Ingredients:

- ◆ 4 **corn tortillas**
- ◆ cooking oil spray
- ◆ 1 tsp. **chili powder**
- ◆ 1 tsp. onion powder
- ◆ 2 tsp. cilantro, dried

Recipe Directions:

Preheat the toaster oven to 450° degrees F. on the bake setting. Line a toaster tray with aluminum foil.

Lightly spray oil onto each side of the tortillas. Stack and cut the corn tortillas into wedges or strips for dipping. Put into a clean plastic bag (gallon size) and sprinkle the spices in. Close and shake until the spices are evenly distributed. Pour out the tortilla chips onto the toaster tray.

Bake in the oven until lightly toasted. Watch these, as they can burn in a second. Remove them when they are almost toasted the way you want them - they will continue to cook outside the oven. Eat when still warm. Leftovers can be saved in an airtight bag. Makes 2 portions.

Nutrition Information:
Calories: 115   Protein: 4 g   Carbs: 24 g   Fat: 1.5 g

Mushroom Bacon Snacks

*Crispy and good, a perfect way to start out
a special dinner with friends*

Ingredients:

♦ 12 large raw mushrooms
♦ 6 slices **bacon** - slices cut in half midway to make 12 pieces
♦ 1/3 cup **barbeque sauce**

Recipe Directions:

Wash mushrooms and dry on a paper towel. Cut the bacon strips in half and wrap a piece of bacon around the mushroom cap. Secure with a toothpick. Place on a foil covered toaster oven pan or greased baking pan. Drizzle the mushrooms with barbeque sauce and roll them around so they are evenly coated.

Bake 15-20 minutes in a 375° degree F oven or until the bacon is crisp. Drizzle with additional barbeque sauce and serve. Makes 4 portions as an appetizer.

Nutrition Information:
Calories: 311   Protein: 9 g   Carbs: 11 g   Fat: 261 g

• • • • • • • • • • • • • • •

Creamy Bean Dip

Use as a dip with fresh vegetables or a flavoring sauce for wraps or steamed vegetables

Ingredients:

- ♦ 3 Tbsp. **hummus bean dip mix, black bean** mix, or **refried bean** mix
- ♦ 1/4 cup hot water
- ♦ 2 Tbsp. **non-dairy or dairy sour cream**
- ♦ 1/4 tsp. **hot pepper sauce**

Recipe Directions:

Mix the bean powder with the hot water. Stir until smooth. Add the sour cream and seasonings to taste. Chill for 1/2 hour for best flavor.

Nutrition Information:
Calories: 99   Protein: 3 g   Carbs: 10 g   Fat: 6 g

S hopping Tip...
Dry bean mixes can be found in the health food sections of many grocery stores as well as food co-ops. Check the label for gluten and dairy free status. They also make a good quick refried bean spread for tacos or quesadillas. Other reasons to like the dry bean mixes... they don't need refrigeration and can be made in small portions.

Spicy Wing Nuts

Fire up study time with a great snack

Ingredients:
- ♦ 2 oz. peanuts (about 1/3 cup)
- ♦ 1 cup **rice checkerboard cereal**
- ♦ 1 cup **puffed rice cereal**
- ♦ 2 Tbsp. **margarine** or substitute
- ♦ 2 Tbsp. hot pepper sauce
- ♦ 1 tsp. **Worcestershire sauce**
- ♦ 1 tsp. rice vinegar or cider vinegar

Recipe Directions:
Preheat the toaster oven to 250° degrees F on the bake setting. Line a toaster oven sheet with aluminum foil.

In a mixing bowl, combine the nuts and the cereals. Heat the butter of margarine in a microwave for 20 seconds. Stir in the pepper sauce, Worcestershire, and vinegar. Heat for another 30 seconds. Pour over the cereal and nut mixture and toss well.

Spread the mixture on the baking sheet and bake for 35-40 minutes, stirring occasionally until crisp. Store in an airtight bag or container. Makes 4 portions.

Nutrition Information:
Calories: 117   Protein: 3 g   Carbs: 8 g   Fat: 9 g

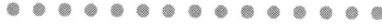

Roasted Chickpeas
A high protein snack for brain power

Ingredients:
- ♦ 1 cup canned **chickpeas**, drained
- ♦ cooking oil spray, olive oil or canola
- ♦ 1/8 tsp. salt
- ♦ 1/4 tsp. **chili pepper**, ground

Recipe Directions:
Preheat oven to 425°F. Place chickpeas on aluminum foil covered baking sheet and spray lightly with olive oil. Sprinkle with salt and chili powder. Roll around to evenly coat. Bake for about 30 minutes, or until golden and crisp. Store leftovers in the refrigerator – warm in microwave or oven. Makes 2 portions.

Nutrition Information...
Calories: 144   Protein: 5 g   Carbs: 27 g   Fat: 1.5 g

Smokin' Pumpkin Seeds

Spice these up as hot as you want with extra seasonings like garlic or red pepper

Ingredients:

- 1 cup pumpkin seeds, raw
- 1 Tbsp. olive or vegetable oil
- 1 tsp. salt
- 1/2 tsp. chili powder
- 1/4 tsp. garlic powder (optional)
- Dash cayenne pepper (optional)

Recipe Directions:

Preheat oven, or toaster oven, to 350° degrees F.

Toss ingredients together in a bowl until well coated. Spread out on an aluminum foil covered baking sheet and bake for 5-7 minutes, or until lightly browned. Remove from oven and allow to cool. Store in an airtight container and use within a week. Makes 4 portions.

Nutrition Information:
Calories: 109   Protein: 4 g   Carbs: 3 g   Fat: 10 g

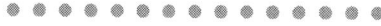

Curried Almonds

A good snack for the back pack

Ingredients:
- ◆ 1 cup whole, raw almonds
- ◆ 2 Tbsp. **margarine** or substitute
- ◆ 1 Tbsp. **curry powder**
- ◆ 1 Tbsp. **Worcestershire sauce**

Microwave Directions:

In a microwave safe 8" round baking dish, place butter or margarine and cook on high for 25 to 40 seconds until melted. Stir in the curry powder and Worcestershire sauce. Add the almonds and stir to coat. Microwave on high for 4 to 5 minutes until almonds are golden brown.

Refrigerate leftovers - they can be re-warmed. Makes 6 portions.

Nutrition Information:
Calories: 129   Protein: 4g   Carbs: 4 g   Fat: 12 g

*V*egan *Friendly...*
Use a dairy free margarine and vegan Worcestershire sauce.

Sweet Sesame Snackers
Easy sweet treat

Ingredients:
- 3/4 cup walnut halves
- 1/8 cup powdered sugar
- 1 1/2 tsp. water
- 2 tsp. sesame seed
- 1/4 tsp. ground cinnamon
- Salt to taste (optional)

Microwave Instructions:
Combine first 3 ingredients in a microwave safe dish, stirring well. Microwave uncovered 1-3 minutes on high. Sugar coating should turn golden brown, not black. Remove from the microwave and stir to coat all the nuts. Sprinkle with sesame seeds, cinnamon and salt. Let the nuts cool completely before eating. If desired, package in small plastic bags for travel around campus. 6 portions.

Nutrition Information...
Calories: 115   Protein: 24 g   Carbs: 51 g   Fat: 102 g

Oatmeal Snack Mix

If your class is in the outback, you will need supplies.

Ingredients:

♦ 2 cups **rolled oats**
♦ 1 sm. bag **coated milk chocolate candy**
♦ 1 snack box raisins
♦ ½ cup **peanuts, dry roasted**, or other nuts

Recipe Directions:

In a toaster oven (or regular oven) set to 300° F. Spread the oatmeal on a toaster oven tray and put in the oven. Stir once or twice as it toasts. Watch the oatmeal until it starts to turn color, about 10 minutes. It should be light brown. Remove from oven and *cool completely*.

In a sealable bag or container, combine all of the ingredients and stir. Store at room temperature. Makes 8 portions.

Note: the candy will melt if it gets too hot, so taking this as a snack during the hot months is not recommended. If it's winter, you're good to go!

Nutrition Information:
Calories: 173   Protein: 5 g   Carbs: 24 g   Fat: 7 g

V egan Friendly...

Substitute a dairy free carob candy for the milk chocolate candy.

• • • • • • • • • • • • • •

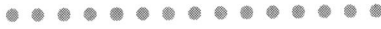

Hot Spinach Dip

What to take to a dorm event...

Ingredients:

- 1 -10 oz. package frozen spinach, defrosted and squeezed dry
- 1 -5.5 oz. can coconut milk
- 4 oz. **soy cheese**, diced; *or* shredded dairy cheese
- 1 small jar diced pimento, drained;
  or 2 Tbsp. diced fresh red pepper
- 1 Tbsp. onion flakes, dehydrated
- 1 1/2 Tbsp. corn starch or potato starch
- 1 tsp. Dijon or yellow **mustard**
- 1 tsp. dill weed, dried
- 1 tsp. **hot pepper sauce**

Rice Cooker Directions:

Squeeze out all the extra water in the defrosted spinach. Mix all the ingredients together in the rice cooker. Turn on to high. Cook for about 12-15 minutes or until the mixture is creamy and thick. Don't stir. Turn cooker to warm setting and serve warm on crackers or vegetable stick dippers. Makes 4 portions

Oven/Toaster Oven Directions:

Preheat the toaster oven to 375°F. Squeeze out the extra water in the defrosted spinach. Mix all the ingredients together in a medium size bowl. Spoon into an oven safe small baking dish or pie plate and smooth out the top. Bake for 15-20 minutes until golden brown.

Nutrition Information...
Calories 157   Protein: 7 g   Carbs: 11 g   Fat: 11g

Hot Spinach Dip, continued

*C*reative Cooking...
 Dip in with gluten free toasted bread, crackers, tortilla
   chips or scoops, or celery and vegetable strips.

Add one can drained and chopped artichoke hearts instead of
the spinach for **Artichoke Dip**, *OR*

Add drained and chopped water chestnuts for crunch.

Add sliced almonds to the top of the dip before baking for a little
decadence.

*S*hopping Tip...
 This is a special occasion dish that can be taken to a group
   meeting or potluck where gluten free foods may be hard to
find. You can take it in the rice cooker and plug it in to keep
warm. Bring along some gluten free dippers and you will be the
hit of the party. Gluten free is good!

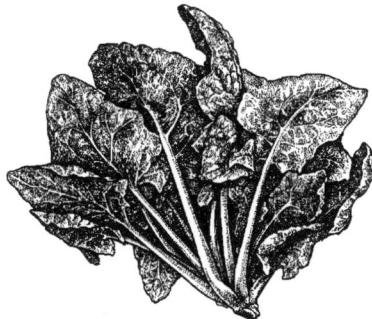

Marshmallow Fondue

Use as a dip for fruit (strawberries, apple slices), an ice cream topping, or chilled as a PB and "fluff" sandwich.

Ingredients:
- ♦   2 cups miniature **marshmallows**
- ♦   2 Tbsp. **rice, soy, almond, or dairy milk**
- ♦   1/2 tsp. **vanilla extract**

Microwave Directions:
In a 1-quart microwave safe container, combine the marshmallows and the milk. Microwave for 40 seconds and stir. Continue in 20-second intervals until the marshmallows are almost melted. Add the vanilla and stir until smooth.

Nutrition Information:
Calories: 322   Protein: 4 g   Carbs: 74 g   Fat: 0.59 g

Creative Cooking...
Add 2 tablespoons jelly or jam at the same time as the vanilla for a fruity dip.

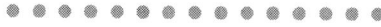

Black Forest Cream

Purchased gluten free biscotti go a long way in this dessert

Ingredients:

- ◆ 1/2 cup **whipped topping** or **dairy free topping**
- ◆ 2 Tbsp. **chocolate syrup**
- ◆ 1 **biscotti cookie,** or other GF cookie
- ◆ 1/4 cup **cherry pie filling**

Recipe Directions:

Combine the defrosted whipped topping with the chocolate syrup. Mix just until combined. Crumble the biscotti into the bottom of a serving dish. Top with the chocolate whip and add cherry pie filling to the top.

Nutrition Information:
Calories: 366   Protein: 4 g   Carbs: 65 g   Fat: 10 g

*L*eftover Tip...
What to do with the leftover cherry pie filling? Make a cobbler by baking or microwaving it in a bowl with a granola or cereal topping mixed with a little sugar and soft margarine or butter. Add nuts if desired. Cook until the topping is crisp.

Chocolate Pudding for One

Gluten free pudding - a treat from the microwave

Ingredients:

- ◆ 1/2 cup **rice, soy, almond or dairy milk**
- ◆ 2 Tbsp. **semi-sweet chocolate chips**
- ◆ 2 tsp. cornstarch; or other thickener like potato starch or arrowroot
- ◆ 1 Tbsp. sugar (approx. 2 sugar packets)

Microwave Directions:

Combine the cornstarch and sugar in a 2-cup microwave safe container. Stir in the milk and chocolate chips. Microwave for 60 to 90 seconds or until hot but not boiling. Stir to melt the chocolate chips.

Continue cooking for 30 to 45 seconds or until the mixture thickens and just begins to boil, or foam. Allow to cool and enjoy warm, or refrigerate for a cold pudding. 1 portion.

Nutrition Information:
Calories: 264   Protein: 6 g   Carbs: 42 g   Fat: 9 g

*C*ooking Tip...
Always combine starches with liquids by putting the starch in the bowl first and then adding the liquid. You will avoid lumps in your final product.

*C*reative Cooking...
You can add all the stir-ins you want. Nuts, other chips, candy bits or pieces, dried fruit like cherries, coconut, or swirl in some fudge topping. Also makes a good chocolate sauce over ice cream when still warm. Have a good time!

Vanilla Pudding
Made simple in a rice cooker...

Ingredients:
- ♦ 1/3 cup sugar, granulated
- ♦ 1/4 cup corn or potato starch
- ♦ 1/4 tsp. salt
- ♦ 1 Tbsp. **margarine** or butter
- ♦ 2 3/4 cups **rice, soy, almond, or dairy milk**
- ♦ 1 tsp. vanilla extract

Rice Cooker Directions:
Combine sugar, corn starch, and salt in rice cooker. Gradually stir in milk until smooth. Stirring constantly with a non-stick spoon or heat resistant spatula, bring to a boil (bubbling) and cook one minute. Turn off and stir in the margarine and vanilla. Pour into serving bowls or into one big bowl. Careful - very hot! Refrigerate. Makes 4 portions.

Nutrition Information...
Calories 205   Protein: 1 g   Carbs: 41 g   Fat: 4 g

*C*reative Cooking...
Add chocolate chips with the margarine and vanilla.
Add dried fruit or coconut at the end of cooking.

Creamy Rice Pudding

What's for dessert? An easy pudding with a creamy texture...

Ingredients:
- 1/2 cup white rice, long grain
- 1/2 cup water
- 3/4 cup apple juice (half a 12 oz. bottle)
- 1 -6 oz. container vanilla **soy** or **dairy yogurt**

Rice Cooker Directions:
Combine rice, water, and apple juice in rice cooker. Turn on and when cooker turns off, remove rice to a bowl. Allow to cool for 10 minutes. Stir in yogurt. Chill. Makes 2 portions.

Stovetop Directions:
Combine rice, water, and apple juice in small saucepan. Turn on to medium heat and cook until all the liquid is absorbed by the rice, remove rice to a bowl. Allow to cool for 10 minutes. Stir in yogurt. Chill. Makes 2 portions.

Microwave Directions:
Combine rice, water, and apple juice in a 2 quart microwave safe container. Cook until rice is tender, about 15-20 minutes, remove rice to a bowl. Allow to cool for 10 minutes. Stir in yogurt. Chill.

Nutrition Information...
Calories: 280   Protein: 6 g   Carbs: 58 g   Fat: 2 g

*C*reative Cooking......
    Add a different flavored yogurt...chocolate, white chocolate
    w/ raspberry, apple and cinnamon, etc. *OR*
Add raisins, dried cranberries, nuts, coconut, or marshmallows.

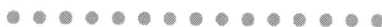

Quick Fruit Dip
Excellent pajama party dip

Ingredients:
- ♦ 1 cup **non-dairy whipped topping**
- ♦ 2 Tbsp. brown sugar
- ♦ 1/4 tsp. cinnamon

Recipe Directions:
In a small bowl, combine the whipped topping, sugar or honey, and cinnamon. Serve as a dip with fruit, especially apple or pear slices.

Nutrition Information:
Calories: 133   Protein: 0.01 g   Carbs: 26 g   Fat: 4 g

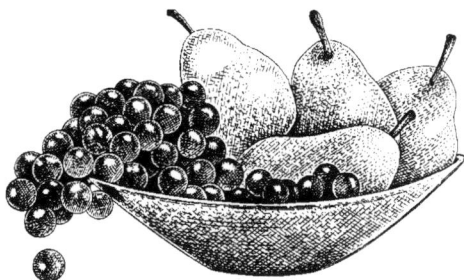

Krispy Peanut Butter Bars

These are "knap sack friendly" for in between classes

Ingredients:
- 1/4 cup sugar
- 1/4 cup pancake syrup, honey, maple or agave syrup
- 1 cup creamy peanut butter, or sun butter
- 1 dash salt
- 2 cups **rice crisp cereal**
- 2/3 cup miniature **marshmallows**

Recipe Directions:
Coat an 8 or 9-inch square or round baking pan with oil or vegetable oil spray, and set aside. A silicone pan works well for this recipe - don't cut the squares while still in the pan - turn out and cut.

To microwave: Combine the sugar, syrup, and salt in a 2-quart microwave safe container. Microwave on high for 3-4 minutes, or until the sugar is dissolved. Blend in peanut butter (or sun butter). Mix until smooth. Immediately add the rice crisp cereal and mini marshmallows. Stir to coat and turn into the greased pan. Press with the back of the spoon until even.

OR

To cook in a saucepan: Combine the sugar, syrup, and salt in a 2 quart saucepan on low heat. Cook and stir until the sugar is dissolved. Blend in peanut butter (or sun butter). Mix until smooth. Immediately add the rice crisp cereal and mini marshmallows. Stir to coat and turn into the greased pan. Press with the back of the spoon until even.

THEN...

Allow to cool for 15 minutes. Cut into squares with a knife dipped in water (this makes it easier to cut). Wrap bars individually with plastic wrap. Store in refrigerator if not eaten within one or two days.

Nutrition Information:
Calories: 284   Protein: 8 g   Carbs: 31 g   Fat: 17 g

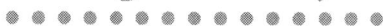

Cocoa Marshmallow Sauce

Serve over ice cream or as a dip with fresh fruit.

Ingredients:

- ♦ 1 1/2 Tbsp. sugar, or alternative sweetener
- ♦ 2 Tbsp. unsweetened cocoa
- ♦ 2 tsp. cornstarch, or other thickener like potato starch
- ♦ 2/3 cup **rice, soy, almond or dairy milk**
- ♦ 2/3 cup miniature **marshmallows**
- ♦ 1 tsp. **vanilla extract**

Recipe Directions:

Measure the cornstarch, sugar and cocoa into a 2-cup microwave safe container. Stir in the milk. Cook on high for 1 minute. Stir. Continue to cook in 20 second intervals and stir well after each round. Depending on the microwave, it will differ how many rounds you will need until your milk mixture starts to thicken. Then add the marshmallows and stir until they are melted. Add the vanilla and stir. Serve hot over ice cream, warm as a dip for fruit, or cold as a spread for toast.

Nutrition Information:
Calories: 125   Protein: 2 g   Carbs: 27 g   Fat: 1 g

*C*reative Cooking...
You can substitute one individual hot cocoa beverage packet for the sugar and cocoa in the recipe. Combine with the cornstarch and follow the rest of the recipe. Flavored hot cocoa mixes will add different flavors to your sauce like chocolate peppermint, chocolate cappuccino, white chocolate, etc. Just make sure the cocoa mix is gluten free!

Screamin' Sandwich

Remember ice cream sandwiches?

Ingredients:
- 1 **frozen waffle**
- ½ cup rice, soy or dairy **chocolate ice cream**
- 1 Tbsp. peanut butter, creamy; or sun butter
- 1 Tbsp. **chocolate syrup**

Recipe Directions:
Toast or reheat gluten free waffle. Cut in half. On one side, drizzle chocolate syrup and on the other spread peanut butter. On the side with the chocolate syrup, spread an even layer of softened ice cream. Top with the other half waffle. Eat now or wrap up to store in the freezer.

Nutrition Information:
Calories: 398   Protein: 7 g   Carbs: 53 g   Fat: 19 g

*C*reative Cooking...
    Well, the combinations are endless. You can use jelly or jam, marshmallow fluff, any nut butter, any GF flavor of ice cream, or any GF syrup or ice cream sauce (like caramel) to upscale your screamin' sandwich. Sprinkle with chopped nuts, mini candies or coconut on the edges.

Crunchy Fruit Cobbler

Enjoy seasonal fruit in a quick dessert from the microwave

Ingredients:
- ♦ 1 medium apple, pear, peach or other fruit
- ♦ 1 1/2 tsp. (1 packet) granulated sugar
- ♦ 1/4 tsp. cinnamon
- ♦ 1/4 cup GF **granola cereal**
- ♦ 1 tsp. **margarine** or substitute

Microwave Directions:
Peel and core the fruit. Slice the fruit in 1/4" thick pieces into a 2-cup microwave safe casserole dish. Sprinkle with the sugar and a dash of cinnamon. Top with granola and dot with butter or margarine. Microwave on 70% power for 4-5 minutes or until the fruit is soft and the top is crunchy. Allow to cool slightly before eating.

Nutrition Information:
Calories: 261   Protein: 5 g   Carbs: 37 g   Fat: 11 g

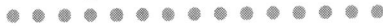

Rice & Fruit Crisp Bars

A small batch for 8 servings.
You don't have to add the fruit to these marshmallow treats,
but it makes them so much more nutritious.
With a mixture of fruits, nuts or seeds, this can be
a great gluten free breakfast bar.

Ingredients:
- ◆   3 cups **crispy brown rice cereal**
- ◆   2 cups miniature **marshmallows**
- ◆   1/2 stick **margarine** or substitute
- ◆   1/2 cup TOTAL dried fruits or other mix-in's – see list

Rice Cooker Directions:
Place rice cereal and your choice of dried fruits, etc. in a large bowl (4 quart). Stir until cereal and add-ins are combined well. Now, melt the margarine in the rice cooker. Add the marshmallows and stir once in a while until the marshmallows are melted. Mix well so the margarine is stirred in.
Pour over the cereal in the bowl and mix with a spatula or non stick spoon. While still warm, press into a non-stick or silicone pan (or greased metal pan). (A cake/pie plate or 8 x8 square pan works well.) Allow to cool completely and cut into bars. Wrap individually in plastic wrap. Store in refrigerator for up to a week, but they won't be around that long! Serves 8

Stovetop Directions:
Place rice cereal and your choice of dried fruits, etc. in a large bowl (4 quart). Stir until cereal and add-ins are combined well. Now, melt the margarine in a 2 quart sauce pan on medium low heat. Add the marshmallows and stir often until the marshmallows are melted. Pull off the heat.
Pour over the cereal in the bowl and mix with a spatula or non-

Rice & Fruit Crisp Bars, continued

stick spoon. While still warm, press into a non-stick or silicone pan (or greased metal pan). (A cake/pie plate or 8" x 8" square pan works well.) Allow to cool completely and cut into bars. Wrap individually in plastic wrap. Store in refrigerator for up to a week, but they won't be around that long! Makes 8 portions.

Microwave Directions:

Place rice cereal and your choice of dried fruits, etc. in a large bowl (4 quart). Stir until cereal and add-ins are combined well. Now, melt the margarine in a 2 quart microwavable container for about one minute. Add the marshmallows and cook for 3-6 minutes until the marshmallows are just melted. Stir so the margarine and marshmallow become blended.

Pour over the cereal in the bowl and mix with a spatula or non stick spoon. While still warm, press into a non-stick or silicone pan (or greased metal pan). (A cake/pie plate or 8 x8 square pan works well.) Allow to cool completely and cut into bars. Wrap individually in plastic wrap. Store in refrigerator for up to a week, but they won't be around that long!

Nutrition Information (with dried fruit)...
Calories 191   Protein: 3 g   Carbs: 26 g   Fat: 9 g

*C*reative Cooking...
Combine your favorite mix-in's to make 1/2 cup total for the recipe...

Raisins
Dried Cranberries
Sunflower Seeds
Pumpkin Seeds
Shredded Coconut
Puffed Amaranth or Flax
Chocolate Chips

More Mini Marshmallows
Dried Banana Chips
Dried Blueberries, Cherries, or Strawberries
Nuts (if allergy tolerant)
Toasted Sesame Seeds
Quinoa Flakes

Exam Chow

*Very addictive...this recipe makes eight servings
so you can share with friends*

Ingredients:

- ◆ 1/2 stick **margarine** or substitute
- ◆ 1/4 cup creamy peanut butter, or sun butter
- ◆ 1 cup **semi-sweet chocolate chips** -about one small package
- ◆ 5 cups **rice checkerboard cereal**
- ◆ 1 cup **mixed nuts**
- ◆ 1 cup powdered sugar (also known as Confectioner's sugar)
- ◆ 1 -2 quart or larger plastic resealable storage bag

Stovetop Directions:

In a large saucepan or skillet, melt the margarine, peanut butter, and chocolate chips on low heat, stirring often. When just melted, remove from heat and stir in the cereal and nuts until well coated. Put into a clean plastic storage bag with the powdered sugar, seal the bag, and toss to coat. You may need additional powdered sugar if it is too sticky. Makes 8 portions.

Microwave Directions:

In a 4-quart microwave safe bowl, melt the margarine, peanut butter, and chocolate chips on 20-second intervals, stirring often. When just melted, stir in the cereal and nuts until well coated. Put into a clean bag with the powdered sugar, seal the bag, and toss to coat. You may need additional powdered sugar if it is too sticky. Makes 8 portions.

Nutrition Information:
Calories: 437   Protein: 7 g   Carbs: 48 g   Fat: 26 g

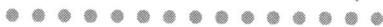

Candy Bar Dessert

Simply the best way to savor the end of the day

Ingredients:

- ♦ 2 *fun size, or 1 small size* gluten free **candy bar**
- ♦ 1 small apple, cored and diced
- ♦ 1/4 cup **non-dairy topping** or whipped cream

Recipe Directions:

Core the apples and cut into small pieces (dice). Cut the candy bars the long way and then make small slices across the two pieces until chopped. Combine the whipped topping, apples, and candy bar. Serve immediately.

Nutrition Information:

Calories: 235   Protein: 3 g   Carbs: 40 g   Fat: 8 g

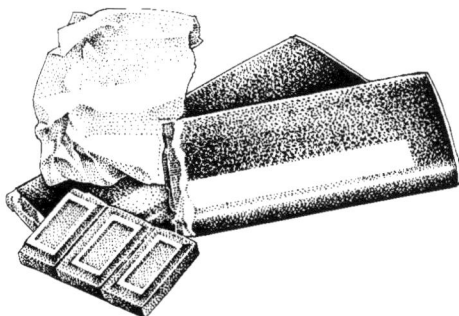

Shaggy Dogs

Missing S'mores? When times get tough, get shaggy!

Ingredients:
- ♦ 8 large **marshmallows**
- ♦ 2 Tbsp. **chocolate syrup**
- ♦ 1/4 cup **rice crisp cereal**

Recipe Directions:
Dip a marshmallow into the chocolate sauce. Immediately dip the chocolate coated marshmallow into the cereal. Roll around. Eat with your fingers and enjoy this sticky mess!

Nutrition Information:
Calories: 228   Protein: 2 g   Carbs: 54 g   Fat: 0.13 g

Chocolate Crisp Candy

Easy way to make your own chocolate crisp candies

Ingredients:
- ♦ 3/4 cup **rice crisp cereal**
- ♦ 1/2 cup **semi-sweet chocolate chips** or vegan chips

Recipe Directions:
Spread the puffed rice out on a toaster oven tray. Toast for 10 minutes at 350° degrees F. While the cereal is warming, microwave the chocolate chips for 25 seconds in a 1 quart microwavable container. Continue microwaving in 10 second intervals until the chips start to look melted – then stir until all the chips are smooth. Pour the toasted cereal into the melted chocolate and stir quickly with a spoon. Drop by the tablespoon full onto a sheet of wax paper or silicone baking sheet. Chill for ½ hour. May be stored covered in the refrigerator for up to a week.

Nutrition Information:
Calories: 120   Protein: 1 g   Carbs: 16 g   Fat: 6 g

*C*reative Cooking...
Substitute 1/4 cup of chopped nuts, dried fruit, *OR* coconut for ¼ cup of rice crisp cereal.

Small Batch Brownies

Lower in fat than many brownies and very simple to make

Ingredients:
- ♦ 1/2 cup cornstarch, or gluten free flour mixture
- ♦ 1/2 cup granulated sugar
- ♦ 3 Tbsp. cocoa, unsweetened dry
- ♦ 1/4 tsp. baking powder
- ♦ 1/8 tsp. salt
- ♦ 3 Tbsp. vegetable oil
- ♦ 1 large egg
- ♦ 2 Tbsp. **chocolate chips**

Recipe Directions:

Note: You will need a small baking pan for this recipe. A bread loaf pan works well, or a small pie pan also is the right size. You can also bake these in a 6 hole muffin pan, filling the muffin tins one half full. Spray with GF cooking oil before putting the batter in the pan.

Preheat oven or toaster oven to 375° F.
Combine all the ingredients in a mixing bowl. Stir until smooth. Spoon into the greased baking pan. If desired, sprinkle with extra chocolate chips. Bake for 20-25 minutes, or until the center is firm and the surface is cracked. Cool. Makes 6 brownies.

Nutrition Information...
Calories: 207   Protein: 1 g   Carbs: 31 g   Fat: 10 g

Beverages

Study tonics for a boost.

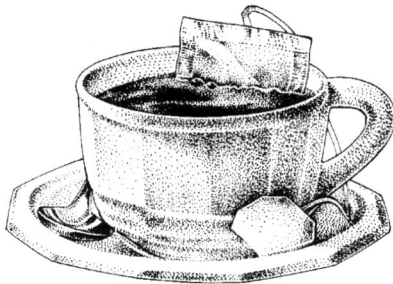

Everywhere you go on campus there are coffee kiosks and quick fill stations for flavored coffees and beverages. Most of them have ingredients you must pass by.

With a little planning, you can order a hot water and stir up your own GF/CF beverage by using one of these mixes. Small reclosable snack bags work great for a portion. Or, mix up a thermal coffee mug for your daily travels. You will also save your spending money for more impressive things.

Note: Items listed in **bold** in the recipes have a higher incidence of containing gluten – it's a *reminder* to always check the label or directly with the manufacturer.

• • • • • • • • • • • • • •

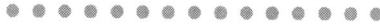

GF/CF Hot Cocoa Mix

Making your own hot cocoa mix is easy,
and easy on the cash flow

Ingredients:

- 2 Tbsp. dairy free milk powder or dairy dry milk powder
- 1 Tbsp. baking cocoa, unsweetened
- 1 1/2 tsp. (1 packet) sugar, granulated
- 1/8 tsp. dry vanilla powder

Recipe Directions:

Mix all ingredients together and store in an airtight bag.
To use: Mix with 1 cup hot water and stir to dissolve.

Nutrition Information:
Calories: 98   Protein: 1 g   Carbs: 23 g   Fat: 2 g

*C*reative Cooking...
You can add dry instant coffee or espresso powder to the
cocoa mix to make a latte flavored drink. Just reduce the
amount of cocoa to your taste.

*S*hopping Tip...
Dry Vanilla Powder can be purchased from gluten free
specialty stores or larger grocery stores.
Dari-free brand dry milk substitute can be used in the beverage
recipes.

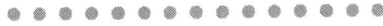

Bulk Size GF/CF Hot Cocoa Mix

Quantity measurements (will make 12 servings):

- 1 1/2 cup dairy free milk powder or other dry milk powder
- 3/4 cup baking cocoa, unsweetened
- 1/3 cup sugar, or equivalent substitute
- 1 1/2 tsp. dry vanilla powder

Combine all ingredients very well. Store in an airtight container and use within 1 month.

To use: Measure 3 tablespoons and combine with 1 cup (8 oz.) hot water.

Nutrition Information:
Calories: 98   Protein: 1 g   Carbs: 23 g   Fat: 2 g

● ● ● ● ● ● ● ● ● ● ● ● ● ● ● ●

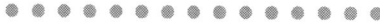

Gluten Free/Casein Free
Sweet Chai Creamer

No need to spend your cash at the coffee house
for a creamy hot chai

Ingredients:
- ♦ 1 Tbsp. dairy free milk powder or other dry milk powder
- ♦ 1 tsp. sugar
- ♦ 1/4 tsp. cinnamon, ground
- ♦ 1/4 tsp. vanilla extract powder

Recipe Directions:
Combine all ingredients and store in an airtight bag.
To use: Stir into hot tea or coffee.
Add-ins: Add a dash of ginger, clove, cardamom, and nutmeg
for a spicy Chai flavor.

Nutrition Information:
Calories: 45   Protein: 0.02 g   Carbs: 11 g   Fat: 0.02 g

Shopping Tip...
Dry Vanilla Powder can be purchased from gluten free
specialty stores or larger grocery stores.
Dari-free brand dry milk substitute can be used in the beverage
recipes

Bulk Size Chai Creamer
(for 12 servings of 1 1/2 Tbsp.)

- ¾ cup dairy free milk powder or other dry milk powder
- 4 Tbsp. sugar
- 1 Tbsp. cinnamon
- 1 Tbsp. dry vanilla powder
- 1/2 tsp. ginger
- 1/2 tsp. clove
- 1/4 tsp. cardamom
- 1/4 tsp. nutmeg

Combine and store in an airtight container for up to one month.

To use: Stir in 1 1/2 tablespoons (about 4 rounded teaspoons) into hot tea or coffee.

Nutrition Information:
Calories: 45   Protein: 0.02 g   Carbs: 11 g   Fat: 0.02 g

Stovetop or Microwave
Vegan Friendly

Study Tonic

Great for colds or as a pick-me-up during long study periods

Ingredients:
- ♦ 2 cups water
- ♦ Juice from 1/2 lemon
- ♦ 2 tsp. honey
- ♦ 5 thin slices raw ginger root

Recipe Directions:

Wash the ginger and cut into chunks (no need to peel). Combine in a bowl or 1-quart container the boiling water, honey, juice from the lemon, and the ginger. Cover and allow to steep for 10 minutes. Strain into a drinking glass. Can also be served over ice like iced tea. Refrigerate leftovers.

This is an excellent drink for times when you need a pick-me-up without caffeine. The fresh ginger is a digestive aid, the honey and lemon will help clear congestion. This drink is perfect when you are not feeling well or just to boost your study concentration.

Nutrition Information:
Calories: 55   Protein: 0.29 g   Carbs: 15 g   Fat: 0.08 g

*S*hopping Tip...

Fresh ginger is excellent for digestion and keeps for quite a while in the refrigerator if wrapped well. Use it in stir fry's or other Asian dishes. It can be found in the produce section and can be purchased by the pound – just buy a small piece to start!

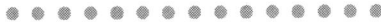

Green Tea Smoothie

You will need a blender or inexpensive beverage mixer
for this recipe

Ingredients:

- ♦ 1 bag green tea
- ♦ 1 cup **rice, soy, almond, or dairy milk**
- ♦ 1 kiwifruit, peeled if desired
- ♦ 1/2 medium banana
- ♦ 2 tsp. **chia seed** (available at health food stores)

Recipe Directions:

Heat the rice or soy milk in a microwave until hot. Steep the tea bag for 5 -10 minutes in the hot milk. In a blender, combine the soy infused milk, the kiwi (washed well and cut into 4 pieces), the banana and the chia seed. Blend until smooth and creamy.

Nutrition Information:
Calories: 275   Protein: 14 g   Carbs: 41 g   Fat: 8 g

*S*hopping Tip...
Chia or salba seeds are available at health food stores, in the health food section of larger grocery stores, and online. These power packed seeds contain amazing protein and nutrition. They also create a feeling of fullness, so if you are keeping the "freshman fifteen" at bay, this morning start is for you.

Microwave and Blender
Vegan Friendly
• • • • • • • • • • • • • • •

Creamy Instant Soup
An economical gluten free alternative to
packaged instant soups

Ingredients:
♦   1 tsp. **chicken** or **vegetable bouillon** (one cube)
♦   2 Tbsp. dry milk powder (Dari free or dairy)
♦   1/2 tsp. parsley flakes
♦   1/4 tsp. onion powder

Recipe Directions:
Combine all ingredients in a mug. Stir in 1 cup very hot water, and cover for 4-6 minutes. Stir again and enjoy.

Make your own instant soup for anywhere on campus. Measure out one recipe into a small zip top bag. Just purchase hot water at a coffee kiosk, stir in, and you will have a quick pick me up.

Nutrient Analysis:
Calories: 90   Protein: 1 g   Carbs: 21 g   Total Fat: 0 g

Gluten Free College Student Cookbook

Breakfast

Pajama perfect starts to the day

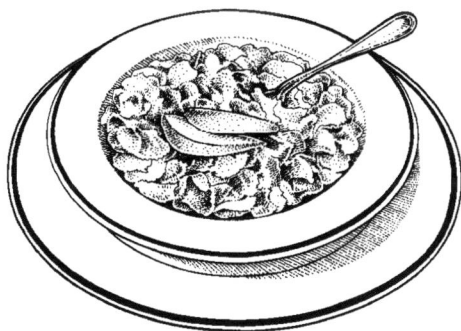

Breakfast Bread Pudding

A warm and syrupy way to start a weekend...

Ingredients:
- ♦ 1/2 cup **rice, soy, almond or dairy milk**
- ♦ 1/2 cup applesauce (1 -4 oz. snack size cup)
- ♦ 1 large egg
- ♦ 1 tsp. brown sugar
- ♦ 2 slices **rice bread**, cubed

Rice Cooker Directions:
Combine the egg, milk, sugar and applesauce in rice cooker. Mix until well combined. Stir in the bread cubes—let the bread absorb the mixture for a couple of minutes. Turn the cooker on and cover. Cook just until the pudding is firm in the center, not runny. Serve with pancake syrup if desired.

Oven/Toaster Oven Directions:
Preheat the oven to 375° F. Combine the egg, milk, sugar and applesauce in a bowl. Mix until well combined. Stir in the bread cubes—let the bread absorb the mixture for a couple of minutes. Dot with margarine or butter. Pour into a greased oven proof 1 quart casserole or bread loaf pan, and bake for 20-25 minutes.

Microwave Directions:
Combine the egg, milk, sugar and applesauce in a microwavable bowl. Mix until well combined. Stir in the bread cubes - let the bread absorb the egg for a couple of minutes. Cover loosely and microwave on high for 3 minutes. Stir once and continue cooking in 30 second intervals until the pudding is firm in the center, not runny. Top with pancake syrup if you like.

Nutrition Information...
Calories 516   Protein: 10 g   Carbs: 80 g   Fat: 18 g

C reative Cooking...
    Spice it up with a dash of cinnamon or nutmeg.
    Add a spoonful of raisins, dried cranberries, or shredded coconut to the mixture before baking.

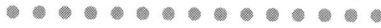

Cheese Strata

The perfect "no classes" brunch dish

Ingredients:

- ♦ 2 slices **bread**, cut into ½" cubes
- ♦ 1/4 cup cubed meltable **soy cheese**,
    or 2 slices Swiss cheese
- ♦ 1 cup **soy or non-dairy creamer**,
    or 1- 8 oz. can evaporated milk
- ♦ 2 large eggs
- ♦ 1 tsp. onion powder
- ♦ 1/2 tsp. dry mustard
- ♦ 1 dash salt
- ♦ 1/8 tsp. black pepper, ground

Recipe Directions:

You will need an 8"x 8" baking pan, or a 3-cup casserole dish for this recipe. Preheat the toaster oven to 350° degrees F. Lightly oil the inside of the dish so the food will release after cooking.

Cube the bread into 1/2" squares. Cut up the cheese slices into small squares about the same size. In a separate mixing bowl, crack the eggs and discard the shells. Stir in the milk, mustard and spices. Add any vegetables if using (see below) and stir in the cheese and bread cubes. Pour mixture into the greased casserole dish. Bake for 25-30 minutes or until the center tests clean. (Cooking Tip...insert the tip of a knife into the center of the casserole, remove it, and if it has no food clinging to it, it is said to test "clean.")
Nutrition Information...
Calories: 413   Protein: 17 g   Carbs: 31 g   Fat: 24g

*C*reative Cooking...

You can add drained canned mushrooms or artichoke hearts, defrosted broccoli pieces, diced onion or peppers, or almost any vegetable that sounds good.
Or try adding diced cooked meat like ham, turkey ham, cooked bacon, smoked turkey, etc.

Scrambled Eggs

Fresh and creamy eggs for anytime of the day...

Ingredients:

- ◆ 2 large eggs
- ◆ 2 tsp. **rice, soy, almond** or dairy milk
- ◆ salt and pepper to taste

Rice Cooker Directions:

Crack eggs into a bowl and add milk. Beat with a fork until well combined. Spray or lightly oil the bottom of the rice cooker. Pour the eggs into the cooker, turn on cook, and stir with a non-stick spoon or spatula until the eggs are cooked the way you like them. Season with salt and pepper to taste.

Microwave Directions:

Crack eggs into a microwave safe bowl and add milk. Beat until well combined. Cover loosely and microwave for 2 minutes on high. Stir and cook in 30 second intervals until done the way you like them. Season with salt and pepper to taste.

Nutrition Information...
Calories: 139   Protein: 7g   Carbs: 1g   Fat: 1 g

Creative Cooking...

Add diced cooked ham, bacon, or sausage, *OR*
Add fresh vegetables like onion, pepper, spinach, diced tomato, etc., *OR*
Add shredded or diced cheese for Cheesy Eggs, *OR*
Add new flavors to breakfast with spices like curry, fajita, or Italian blends. Start with ¼ teaspoon and work your way up.

Shopping Tip...

If you are tolerant of eggs, hard boiled eggs make great travel lunches when away from gluten free dining areas. Just remember to pack them in a cooler bag and eat promptly.

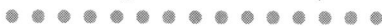

Crunchy Granola

A less expensive way to have granola everyday

Ingredients:

- ♦ 1 cup **rolled oats** (check gluten free status)
- ♦ 1/3 cup walnuts, chopped
- ♦ 1/4 cup **rice bran**
- ♦ 2 Tbsp. brown sugar, packed
- ♦ 2 Tbsp. honey
- ♦ 1/2 tsp. vanilla extract
- ♦ 1/2 tsp. cinnamon, ground
- ♦ 1 snack box raisins
- ♦ 2 Tbsp. coconut

Recipe Directions:

In a microwave safe baking dish, combine the oats, nuts, rice bran, and brown sugar. In a small bowl, mix together the honey, vanilla extract, and cinnamon. Pour over the oat mixture and stir well. Microwave on high for 3 to 5 minutes, or until hot, stirring 2 or 3 times. Stir in raisins and coconut. Store in a covered container. Makes 4 portions.

Nutrition Information:
Calories: 246   Protein: 5 g   Carbs: 38 g   Fat: 10 g

CreativeCooking...

Add dried fruits like banana chips, diced dried tropical fruit, different nuts and seeds, or small amounts of chocolate chips after cooking for a real trail mix cereal.

Yogurt Parfait

Good for a lunch on the go or a library snack.
Just be sure to use a well-chilled thermal container and eat
within 2-3 hours of taking it out of the refrigerator.

Ingredients:

- 1 -6 oz. container **soy or dairy vanilla yogurt**
- 1/2 cup applesauce (1- 4 oz. individual portion cup)
- 1/4 cup **rice crisp cereal**

Recipe Directions:

In a water glass or other container, layer the yogurt, applesauce, and cereal. Finish with the cereal, or add nuts if tolerant. Enjoy. Makes 1 portion.

Nutrition Information:
Calories: 257   Protein: 7 g   Carbs: 54 g   Fat: 3 g

*C*reative Cooking...

Try different flavors of yogurt with different flavors of applesauce.
Sprinkle in dried fruits instead of cereal, especially tropical fruit bits or coconut.
Use trail mix or a gluten free granola instead of breakfast cereal.

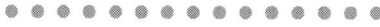

Baked Potato Hash Browns

The leftover baked potato goes uptown in three versions of breakfast potatoes

Ingredients:
♦ 1 baked potato
♦ 1 tsp. **margarine** or substitute
♦ 1 tsp. dried minced onion
♦ 1/2 tsp. garlic powder
♦ 1/2 tsp. paprika

Recipe Directions:
Cut the leftover cooked baked potato into slices, cubes or wedges. Heat the margarine in a pan (or rice cooker) adding the potatoes, onion flakes (or fresh diced onion), garlic powder and paprika. As the potatoes get hot, move them around with a non-stick spoon or turner. When the potatoes are nicely browned, they are ready for eating.

Nutrition Information:
Calories: 175   Protein: 4 g   Carbs: 32 g   Fat: 4 g

Creative Cooking...
Ranch Potatoes: Instead of the onion flakes and garlic powder, sprinkle about 1/2 to 1 teaspoon ranch seasoning mix on the potatoes. Cook according to the recipe.

Barbeque Potatoes: When potatoes are browned, add about one tablespoon barbeque sauce and stir quickly. Serve.

Tropical Quinoa
A filling hot breakfast cereal with a nutritional punch

Ingredients:
- ♦ 1/3 cup quinoa flakes
- ♦ 1/4 tsp. ground cinnamon
- ♦ 3 Tbsp. **dried tropical fruit mix**
- ♦ 2/3 cup water

Rice Cooker Directions:
Combine all ingredients in the rice cooker. Turn on, cover and cook until the rice cooker turns to warm setting. Add 1 tablespoon of water and allow to rest covered for 3 minutes on the warm. Stir and eat.

Stovetop Directions:
Combine all ingredients in a small saucepan on medium heat. Turn on, cover and cook until the quinoa is thick about 5-7 minutes. Stir occasionally.

Microwave Directions:
Combine mix and water in microwave safe container. Cover loosely and cook for 2 minutes. Stir and continue to cook in 15 second increments until thick. Cool slightly before eating.

Nutrition Information...
Calories: 247   Protein: 6 g   Carbs: 49 g   Fat: 4 g

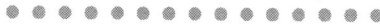

Stomach Soothing Congee

Congee is a thin rice porridge traditionally eaten in Asian countries for breakfast. It also takes several hours to cook. Here is a stomach-soothing version for sick days that you can cook quickly and spice up to your tastes.

Ingredients:
♦ 1/4 cup white rice
♦ 2 1/2 cups water
♦ 1/2 tsp. **vegetable or chicken bouillon** (1/2 cube)

Recipe Directions:
In a small saucepan or rice cooker, combine all the ingredients and bring to a boil. Turn to simmer and allow the rice to cook until very soft, about 30 minutes. Mash with a potato masher or blend (careful of hot liquids). Broth should be thin and lightly cloudy from the dissolved rice.

Nutrition Information:
Calories: 175   Protein: 4 g   Carbs: 37 g   Fat: 1 g

*C*reative Cooking...
Add cooked meats like chicken or turkey, soy sauce or tamari, fresh ginger, or a dash of sesame oil. You can also add almost any vegetables (diced small) in the last 5 minutes of cooking.

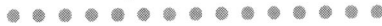

Basic Waffle Mix

*If you love waffles and have a waffle maker,
these will save on your food budget*

Ingredients:

- 1 3/4 cup gluten free flour mix (*or* 1 cup white rice flour, 1/2 cup potato starch, and 1/4 cup tapioca flour)
- 2 tsp. **baking powder**
- 1 tsp. salt
- 1/4 cup vegetable oil
- 2 large eggs
- 1 1/4 cup **rice, soy, almond, or dairy milk**
- 1 Tbsp. sugar (about 2 packets of sugar)
- 1 tsp. vanilla extract
- 1 tsp. cinnamon, ground

Recipe Instructions:

Turn on the waffle maker to warm up.

Crack the eggs into a medium bowl and mix until one color. Add the rest of the ingredients and stir. The batter should be smooth. The thickness of the batter can be adjusted by adding a little more milk. You want a batter that flows easily over the waffle grid, but not so runny that it won't stay in the waffle iron.

Use your one cup measure and scoop up a cup of the batter. Use just enough of the batter to fill the lower waffle grid but not flow over. Put the lid down and let the waffle cook until crisp and golden brown. Use the remaining batter for 1 and a half more waffles in a standard small waffle maker. Each waffle is a serving for most people, two is a big meal. Wrap and freeze the extra waffles.

Nutrition Information...
Calories: 367   Protein: 7 g   Carbs: 52 g   Fat: 14 g

Salads

Crunchy and good – back pack friendly too

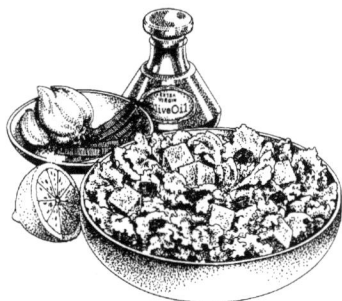

So you eat a lot of salads everywhere you go because that's what's gluten free at many food venues. Here are some interesting salads that you might not find out and about, but are also healthy dorm snacks.

If you're on a budget, filling up a thermal carrier with your lunch or dinner is a good way to avoid cross contamination and save a few dollars.

Note: Items listed in **bold** in the recipes have a higher incidence of containing gluten – it's a *reminder* to always check the label or directly with the manufacturer.

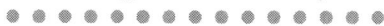

Crunchy Fruit Salad

This salad is satisfyingly crunchy. Add some nuts or sunflower seeds for added protein.

Ingredients:
- ♦ 1 small apple, cored and diced
- ♦ 1 small banana, sliced
- ♦ 1 small stalk celery, sliced
- ♦ 1 small bunch green grapes, cut in half if desired
- ♦ 1/4 cup **vanilla soy yogurt, or dairy yogurt**

Recipe Directions:
Combine all fruit and the celery in a small bowl. Add the yogurt and stir to coat the fruit. Top with nuts if desired. Makes 1 portion.

Nutrition Information:
Calories: 239   Protein: 4 g   Carbs: 58 g   Fat: 2 g

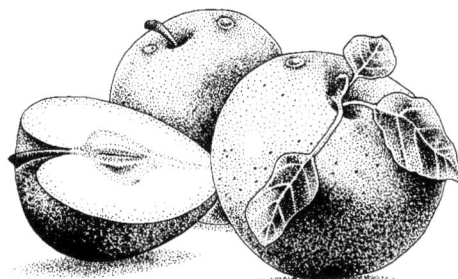

Chinese Chicken Salad

Try this salad with marinated tofu instead of chicken

Ingredients:

- ♦ 1 -5 oz. can **chicken**, drained; *or* 1/3 cup **cooked chicken**
- ♦ 2 cups Chinese or Napa cabbage, shredded
- ♦ 1 -6 oz. can mandarin orange segments, well drained
- ♦ 2 Tbsp. canola oil
- ♦ 2 Tbsp. rice vinegar
- ♦ 1/2 packet sugar
- ♦ 1 tsp. **soy sauce or tamari**
- ♦ 2 Tbsp. **peanuts, dry roasted** (optional)

Recipe Directions:

Drain the juice from the mandarin oranges. Cut the cabbage in fine strips. Drain the chicken and add to the bowl with the cabbage and mandarin oranges. In a separate small bowl, combine the oil, vinegar, sugar and soy sauce or tamari. Pour over the salad and lightly toss with a fork. Top with the peanuts. Makes 2 portions.

Nutrition Information:
Calories: 358   Protein: 17 g   Carbs: 21 g   Fat: 24 g

Honey Mustard Apple Salad

Very quick and easy with leftover cooked rice

Ingredients:
- ♦ 1/2 cup white rice, *cooked*
- ♦ 1 small apple, cored and diced
- ♦ 2 Tbsp. **honey mustard salad dressing**
- ♦ 1 Tbsp. raisins

Recipe Directions:
Dice the apple into 1/2" cubes. Toss with the salad dressing and then add the rice and raisins. Chill.

Nutrition Information:
Calories: 333   Protein: 3 g   Carbs: 51 g   Fat: 14 g

C reative Cooking...
Add your favorite nuts, dried fruits, or diced chicken or turkey.

Warm Potato Salad

A microwaved potato becomes a center stage salad

Ingredients:
- ♦ 1 baked potato
- ♦ 2 tsp. rice vinegar
- ♦ 1 packet sugar
- ♦ 1 tsp. olive oil
- ♦ 1 Tbsp. **bacon bits**

Recipe Directions:
Microwave or bake a potato until cooked. Allow to cool for 10 minutes. In a small bowl, combine the vinegar, sugar, and oil. Cube the warm potato into 1/2" square pieces. Stir into the dressing and sprinkle the bacon bits over the top. Makes 1 portion.

Nutrition Information:
Calories: 220   Protein: 6 g   Carbs: 35 g   Fat: 6 g

C **reative Cooking...**
Alternatives for the bacon include: sunflower seeds, shredded cheese, marinated tofu, or chopped nuts. Also good with honey mustard dressing instead of the oil and vinegar dressing.

Mexi-corn Salad

*Crunchy corn salad to go with anything Mexican,
or on its own*

Ingredients:
- ♦ 1 -8 oz. can Mexican corn, drained
- ♦ 2 Tbsp. **Italian salad dressing**
- ♦ about 12 corn chips, crushed

Recipe Directions:
Drain the corn well. Combine the corn, salad dressing, and crumbled corn chips. Serve. Makes 1 large portion.

Nutrition Information:
Calories: 354   Protein: 7 g   Carbs: 48 g   Fat: 14 g

C reative Cooking...
Experiment with adding sunflower seeds, black olives from a deli, salsa instead of salad dressing, or cooked grains like quinoa or rice (adjust the dressing to taste).

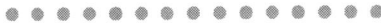

Orange Quinoa Salad

Great for a traveling lunch in a thermal container

Ingredients:
- ♦ 1/3 cup quinoa, *cooked*
- ♦ 2 Tbsp. **raspberry vinaigrette salad dressing**
- ♦ 1 -4 oz. snack size mandarin oranges, drained
- ♦ 1 Tbsp. almonds, sliced

Recipe Directions:
Combine the cooked quinoa (or rice) with the drained mandarin oranges, the salad dressing, and the almonds. Makes 1 portion.

Nutrition Information:
Calories: 333   Protein: 7 g   Carbs: 56 g   Fat: 10 g

*C*ooking Tip...

To Cook an individual portion of Quinoa:

Microwave: Combine 1/3 cup washed quinoa with 2/3 cup water in a 2-cup microwave dish. Cover lightly and microwave on full power for 4-6 minutes.

Rice Cooker or Stovetop: Combine 1/3 cup washed quinoa with 2/3 cup water in the cooker or pan on stove. Cook covered on medium heat for 10-12 minutes, turn off heat and allow to rest for 5 minutes.

Condiments and
Dressings

Spicin' it up is easy to do

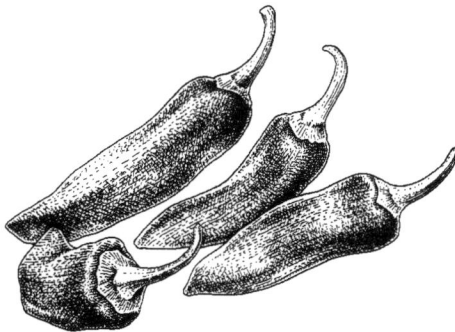

The thing about learning to cook is that you find out how easy it is to make many packaged foods. You also find out that it's so much less expensive to *do it yourself.* The time it takes is often less than the time it takes to go going shopping. It's also much safer to know that the gluten contamination issue is under your control.

In this section, there are recipes for condiments, dressings, and seasonings that will make your gluten free life easier. Once you get the hang of putting foods together, you'll never look back.

Note: Items listed in **bold** in the recipes have a higher incidence of containing gluten – it's a *reminder* to always check the label or directly with the manufacturer.

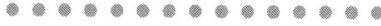

Chicken Gravy

Gluten Free/Dairy Free gravy for mashed potatoes and meats

Ingredients:

- ♦ 1 cup water
- ♦ 1 cube **chicken bouillon**; or **vegetable bouillon**
- ♦ 1 Tbsp. **margarine** or substitute
- ♦ 2 Tbsp. cornstarch, or potato starch
- ♦ 1/4 tsp. sage or **poultry seasoning**
- ♦ 1 dash black pepper

Stovetop Directions:

In a small saucepan, heat the water, bouillon and margarine until boiling. In a small bowl, combine the cornstarch or potato starch with 3 tablespoons water. Add to the gravy, stirring constantly. Add the pepper and sage. Cook on simmer for 3-4 minutes.

Microwave Directions:

Combine all ingredients. Cook/stir in 30 second intervals until the gravy is thick.

Nutrition Information:
Calories: 105   Protein: 0.01 g   Carbs: 14 g   Fat: 6 g

Southwest Salad Dressing or Dip

Use as a salad dressing for taco salad, as a quick nacho dip, or with vegetables.

Ingredients:
- ♦ 1/3 cup salsa
- ♦ 2 Tbsp. **non-dairy or dairy sour cream**
- ♦ 1 ½ tsp. granulated sugar (1 packet)

Recipe Directions:
Combine all ingredients and chill. Makes 2 portions.

Nutrition Information:
Calories: 61   Protein: 0.50 g   Carbs: 10 g   Fat: 4 g

Stir Fry Thickening Sauce

Add to stir-fry when the vegetables and meats are almost done.
It will thicken, glaze and season your stir-fry.

Ingredients:
- ♦ 1 tsp. cornstarch (or 1 ½ tsp. potato starch)
- ♦ 1/4 cup water
- ♦ 1 tsp. **soy sauce or tamari**
- ♦ 1/2 tsp. toasted **sesame oil**

Recipe Directions:
Measure the cornstarch into a liquid measuring cup. Add water to the 1/4 cup line. Add the soy sauce or tamari, sesame oil, and seasonings. Stir well. Enough for a one person stir fry – can be doubled or tripled.

To use: Add the sauce at the last 2-3 minutes of cooking time when stir frying meats or vegetables. Cook until glossy and clear.

Nutrition Information:
Calories: 35   Protein: 1 g   Carbs: 3 g   Fat: 2 g

Honey Mustard I

It doesn't get easier than this for a great dipping sauce

Ingredients:
- ♦ 1 Tbsp. honey
- ♦ 1 Tbsp. **Dijon** or **prepared mustard**

Recipe Directions:
Mix together and use as a dipping sauce or salad dressing.
Makes 1 portion.

Nutrition Information:
Calories: 75   Protein: 0.00 g   Carbs: 20 g   Fat: 0.00 g

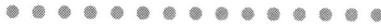

Honey Mustard II

There is added flavor in this creamy version of a
very versatile sauce or salad dressing

Ingredients:

- 2 Tbsp. mayonnaise
- 1 Tbsp. honey
- 1 Tbsp. **Dijon** or **prepared mustard**
- 1/4 tsp. **Worcestershire sauce**
- 1/4 tsp. onion powder

Recipe Directions:

Mix together until smooth. Use as a dipping sauce or salad dressing. Makes 2 portions.

Nutrition Information:
Calories: 93   Protein: 0.02 g   Carbs: 7 g   Fat: 7 g

Chili con Carne Spice

This recipe will flavor about 3 small batches of chili.
Spice mixes are great gifts from home.

Ingredients:

- 2 Tbsp. chili powder
- 1 1/2 Tbsp. cumin, ground
- 1 Tbsp. onion flakes
- 1 Tbsp. ground coriander, or dried cilantro
- 1 Tbsp. garlic powder
- 1 Tbsp. paprika
- 1 tsp. crushed red pepper
- 1 tsp. oregano
- 1/2 tsp. black pepper, ground
- 1/2 tsp. allspice, ground
- 1/4 tsp. cayenne pepper (optional)

Recipe Directions:

Combine all spices in an airtight container. Use 3 tablespoons (or more to taste) for a quart of chili (about 4 servings). Enough mix for 3 batches of chili.

Nutrition Information:
Calories: 8   Protein: 0.33 g   Carbs: 1 g   Fat: 0.30 g

Quick Chili

Brown ½ lb. cooked (browned and drained) ground beef, turkey, or chicken in a large saucepan or rice cooker. Drain. Add one can diced tomatoes, one can tomato sauce, one can drained red kidney beans, and 2-4 Tbsp. of the chili seasoning. Bring to a boil and simmer for 20-30 minutes.

No Cook
Vegan Friendly

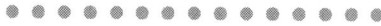

• • • • • • • • • • • • • • • •

Ranch Seasoning Mix

The king of GF/CF dressings and dips.
This mix would be a great gift in a care package from home.

Ingredients:

- ♦   1/4 cup parsley flakes
- ♦   2 Tbsp. dried minced onion
- ♦   2 Tbsp. onion powder
- ♦   1 Tbsp. garlic powder
- ♦   2 tsp. garlic salt
- ♦   1 Tbsp. potato starch or cornstarch
- ♦   1 tsp. dill weed
- ♦   1/2 tsp. marjoram
- ♦   1/2 tsp. celery seed

Recipe Directions:

Combine all ingredients in an air tight container for up to six months. Optional – Pulse in a blender or food processor to combine well.

Nutrition Information for 1 teaspoon mix:
Calories: 20   Protein: 0.43 g   Carbs: 4 g   Fat: 0.06 g

To make dressing: Combine one teaspoon mix with 1/4 cup mayonnaise, 1/4 cup sour cream or substitute, and 2 tablespoons milk or milk substitute. Mix well and chill for one hour. Thin with additional milk to get desired consistency for dip or salad dressing. Use within 4 days.

C reative Cooking...
The dry seasoning mix may also be used dry to flavor potatoes, vegetables, pasta, or other foods. Be creative!

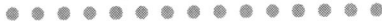

Pizza Seasoning

Use on pizza or in any Italian style pasta, casserole, or soup

Ingredients:
- ♦ 2 Tbsp. oregano
- ♦ 1 1/2 Tbsp. basil
- ♦ 1 Tbsp. marjoram
- ♦ 2 tsp. granulated garlic
- ♦ 1/2 tsp. crushed red pepper

Recipe Directions:
Combine all ingredients and keep in an airtight container for up to 6 months. Use on pizza, pasta, or in Italian main dishes.

Nutrition Information for 1 teaspoon mix:
Calories: 6   Protein: 0.21 g   Carbs: 1 g   Fat: 0.07 g

Taco Seasoning

Flavor tacos, nachos, wraps, or casseroles with this all-purpose Mexican seasoning

Ingredients:

- ♦   6 Tbsp. chili powder
- ♦   5 Tbsp. paprika
- ♦   4 Tbsp. cumin, ground
- ♦   3 Tbsp. onion powder
- ♦   1 Tbsp. garlic powder
- ♦   5 Tbsp. cornstarch or potato starch

Recipe Directions:

Combine all spices and store in an airtight container.
Makes 12- two tablespoon servings.

Nutrition Information for 1 tablespoon mix:
Calories: 26   Protein: 0.79 g   Carbs: 5 g   Fat: 1 g

*H*ow to use···
Use 2 Tablespoons taco seasoning with 1/2 pound of browned ground meat (or crumbled tofu), and one small can of tomato sauce for quick taco meat. Heat to bubbling. Makes 2-3 portions.

All Purpose Seasoning
Use it in just about everything

Ingredients:
- 1 1/2 tsp. sage, ground
- 1 tsp. paprika
- 1 tsp. garlic powder
- 1 tsp. onion powder
- 3/4 tsp. thyme, dried
- 1/2 tsp. black pepper, ground
- 1/2 tsp. marjoram, dried
- 1/2 tsp. rosemary, ground
- 1/4 tsp. nutmeg, ground
- 1 tsp. salt (optional)

Recipe Instructions:
Combine all ingredients. Optional - pulse in a blender. Store in an air-tight container.

Use a 1/2 teaspoon of this seasoning to boost the flavor of soups, stews, sauces, dips, dressings and casseroles.

Nutrition Information for ½ teaspoon mix:
Calories: 4   Protein: 1 g   Carbs: 2 g   Fat: 0 g

S hopping Tip:
I encourage you to learn about spices, but if this is too many different spices to keep in your dorm kitchen, consider making this mix at home on break. Feel free to change it to your tastes.

Simple Curry Powder

If you can't find a gluten free curry powder, this simple recipe will give you that curry flavor in any recipe

Ingredients:

- ♦ 2 Tbsp. cumin, ground
- ♦ 2 Tbsp. coriander, ground
- ♦ 2 tsp. turmeric, ground
- ♦ 1 tsp. red pepper, crushed flakes
- ♦ 1/2 tsp. dry mustard, ground (this is the dry spice, not the prepared mustard)
- ♦ 1/2 tsp. ginger, ground (also the dry spice, not the fresh root)

Recipe Instructions:

Combine all spices and store in an air tight container. Optional – grind in a blender or small food processor.

Use 1/4 to 1/2 teaspoon per one serving.

Nutrition Information for ½ teaspoon mix:
Calories: 14   Protein: 1 g   Carbs: 2 g   Fat: 1 g

Shopping Tip...

Curry powder is really a mixture of eight or more spices and can come in many different colors and degrees of heat. Although wheat flour is rarely used in Indian cooking, always check that it is from a gluten free manufacturer.

Creole Spice

*More flavor than heat in this seasoning for adding
a New Orleans spice to your cooked foods*

Ingredients:
- ♦ 1 tsp. cayenne pepper
- ♦ 1 tsp. basil, dried
- ♦ 1 tsp. oregano, dried
- ♦ 1/2 tsp. black pepper, ground
- ♦ 1/2 tsp. thyme, dried
- ♦ 1/2 tsp. garlic powder

Mix all ingredients and store in an air-tight container. Use ¼ to ½ teaspoon as a seasoning to taste. Excellent as a rub to coat meats, fish and poultry before cooking. Gives soups and stews a slightly spicy flavor without being too hot. Makes about 12 servings.

Nutrition Information for ½ teaspoon mix:
Calories: 3   Protein: 0 g   Carbs: 1 g   Fat: 0 g

Hot Stuff

If you love spicy food, this will wake up your taste buds.
Try it on beef, chicken, pork, or tofu

Ingredients:

♦   3 Tbsp. chili powder
♦   1 1/2 tsp. garlic powder
♦   2 tsp. ground cumin
♦   1 tsp. oregano
♦   1/2 tsp. red chili flakes
♦   1 packet sugar, granulated

Recipe Instructions:

Combine all ingredients and store in an airtight container.
Shake before using to blend. To apply the rub, simply cover the
outside surface of the meat with the seasoning blend before
cooking. The heavier the coating, the spicier it will be! Makes 16
portions.

Nutrition Information for ½ teaspoon of mix:
Calories: 15   Protein: 1 g   Carbs: 3 g   Fat: .5 g

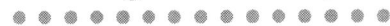

Oriental Seasoning
A quick fix to rice or stir fry

Ingredients:
- 2 Tbsp. minced onion
- 2 Tbsp. ginger, ground
- 2 Tbsp. garlic powder
- 2 tsp. black pepper, ground
- 1 Tbsp. **gomasio** (sesame salt), or 2 Tbsp. sesame seeds

Recipe Directions:
Combine all ingredients in an airtight container or bag for up to 6 months. Use ½ teaspoon to season a dish for 1-2 people.

Nutrient Analysis:
Calories: 10   Protein: 1 g   Carbs: 2 g   Total Fat: 1 g

*S*hopping Tip···
Gomasio is a sesame seed salt that can be found in many health food stores or in an Asian foods section of a grocery store. You can substitute toasted or regular sesame seeds and add a little salt to the mix if desired.

Quesadillas and Tostadas

Fire up some South of the Border food in a flash

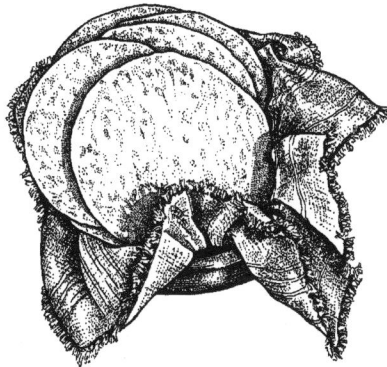

Tips for making gluten free quesadillas:

You can use corn tortillas, brown rice wraps, or teff wraps for quesadillas. The size of these wraps will vary greatly, so please work with the instructions in the recipes and the amounts according to which size you are using. Gluten free wraps are much more pliable when they are heated. If you have trouble folding the larger wraps, cut one in half and use each side as a tortilla.

Besides a skillet, you can also use an electric fry pan, a clam shell sandwich grill (think Forman), or microwave for making great quesadillas. Simply heat the skillet to medium and lay a lightly buttered gluten free wrap in the pan. Add the fillings and another wrap (buttered side up). Heat until the bottom wrap is lightly brown and the fillings start to melt together. Flip over and brown on the other side. Slide out onto a plate and cut into wedges.

If you are using the large gluten free brown rice or teff wraps, this will feed two people easily (or ONE *very well*). For a smaller portion, you can use one wrap in the pan, spread out the filling, and fold together when the fillings have started to melt. Brown on each side.

When using meltable soy cheese and grilling in a skillet, sometimes the wrap does not get hot enough to melt the cheese without burning. You may want to grill for the nice brown outer surface and then slide onto a plate and cook in the microwave for $\frac{1}{2}$ to 1 minute to thoroughly melt the cheese.

What to fill a quesadilla with? Here are some excellent fillings to get you started as a master gluten free quesadilla artist.

Note: Items listed in **bold** in the recipes have a higher incidence of containing gluten – it's a **reminder** to always check the label or directly with the manufacturer.

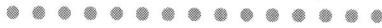

Taco Quesadilla
A side of salsa for dipping makes this dish complete

Ingredients:
- ♦ 1 gluten free tortilla wrap
- ♦ 1 tsp. **margarine** or butter
- ♦ 2 oz. (or ¼ cup) taco meat (beef, turkey, chicken or tofu) - recipe on page 239
- ♦ 1 oz. (or 1/8 cup) meltable **soy cheese** or dairy cheese
- ♦ 2 Tbsp. salsa
- ♦ 2 tsp. canned jalapeno pepper rings (optional)
- ♦ 4 black olives, chopped (optional)

Stovetop Instructions:
Heat a 12" "skillet on medium heat. Lightly butter one side of a tortilla wrap and place the buttered side down on the skillet. Evenly spread the cheese, taco meat, salsa, and condiments over half the tortilla – fold over the empty side. Continue cooking until the bottom of the tortilla starts to brown. Flip the tortilla over with a spatula and brown the other side. Quesadilla is done when the filling is hot and the outside is golden brown. Makes 1 portion.

Microwave Instructions:
Thinly spread margarine or butter on the wrap and place butter side down on a paper towel. Layer the cheese, taco meat, salsa, and condiments on the tortilla. Microwave on the paper towel on high power for 1 ½ to 2 minutes, or until the fillings are hot and the cheese melted. Allow to cool slightly, fold over in half, and cut into wedges. Makes 1 portion.

Nutrition Information...
Calories: 521   Protein: 26 g Carbs: 39 g   Fat: 28 g

Stovetop or Microwave
Vegan Friendly
● ● ● ● ● ● ● ● ● ● ● ● ● ●

Honey Mustard Chicken Quesadilla
Wake up your taste buds

Ingredients:
- ♦ 1 gluten free tortilla wrap
- ♦ 1 tsp. **margarine** or substitute
- ♦ 6 slices **deli turkey breast** (or **seasoned tofu slices**)
- ♦ 1 oz. (or 1/8 cup) meltable **soy cheese** or dairy cheese
- ♦ 2 tsp. **honey mustard**

Stovetop Directions:
Heat a skillet on medium heat. Lightly butter one side of a tortilla wrap and place the buttered side down on the skillet. Evenly spread the cheese, turkey (or tofu) and honey mustard over half the tortilla – fold over the empty side. Continue cooking until the bottom of the tortilla starts to brown. Flip the tortilla over with a spatula and brown the other side. The quesadilla is done when the filling is hot and the outside is golden brown. Makes 1 portion.

Microwave Instructions:
Thinly spread margarine or butter on the wrap and place buttered side down on a paper towel. Layer the cheese, turkey (or tofu) and honey mustard on the tortilla. Microwave on the paper towel on high power for 1 ½ to 2 minutes, or until the fillings are hot and the cheese melted. Allow to cool slightly, fold over in half, and cut into wedges. Makes 1 portion.

Nutrition Information...
Calories: 441   Protein: 17 g   Carbs: 34 g   Fat: 25 g

Turkey Taco Quesadilla

Spice up a turkey sandwich into an event

Ingredients:

- 1 gluten free tortilla wrap
- 1 tsp. vegetable oil or **margarine**
- 2 Tbsp. salsa or guacamole
- 2 oz. **deli turkey breast** (or **seasoned tofu slices**)
- 1 oz. (or 1/8 cup) meltable **soy cheese** or alternative
- 1/4 tsp. **taco seasoning mix**

Stovetop Instructions:

Heat a skillet on medium heat. Lightly butter one side of a tortilla wrap and place the buttered side down on the skillet. Evenly spread the salsa, turkey (or tofu), cheese, and taco seasoning over half the tortilla – fold over the empty side. Continue cooking until the bottom of the tortilla starts to brown. Flip the tortilla over with a spatula and brown the other side. It is done when the filling is hot and the outside is golden brown. Makes 1 portion.

Microwave Instructions:

Thinly spread margarine or butter on the wrap and place butter side down on a paper towel. Layer the salsa, turkey (or tofu), cheese, and taco seasoning on the tortilla. Microwave on the paper towel on high power for 1 ½ to 2 minutes, or until the fillings are hot and the cheese melted. Allow to cool slightly, fold over in half, and cut into wedges. Makes 1 portion.

Nutrition Information...
Calories: 428   Protein: 19 g   Carbs: 35 g   Fat: 22 g

Bean and Rice Quesadilla
Add sour cream or guacamole for extra rich flavor

Ingredients:
- ♦ 1 gluten free tortilla wrap
- ♦ 1 tsp. **margarine** or substitute
- ♦ 3 Tbsp. **refried beans**
- ♦ 1/2 cup *cooked* **Spanish** or other **flavorful rice** (see quick recipe on pg. 218)
- ♦ 1 oz. (or 1/8 cup) meltable **soy cheese** or Jack cheese
- ♦ 2 Tbsp. salsa

Stovetop Instructions:
Heat a skillet on medium heat. Lightly butter one side of a tortilla wrap and place the buttered side down on the skillet. Evenly spread the beans, rice, cheese, and salsa over half the tortilla – fold over the empty side. Continue cooking until the bottom of the tortilla starts to brown. Flip the tortilla over with a spatula and brown the other side. It is done when the filling is hot and the outside is golden brown. Makes 1 portion.

Microwave Instructions:
Thinly spread margarine or butter on the wrap and place butter side down on a paper towel. Layer the beans, rice, cheese, and salsa on the tortilla. Microwave on the paper towel on high power for 1 ½ to 2 minutes, or until the fillings are hot and the cheese melted. Allow to cool slightly, fold over in half, and cut into wedges. Makes 1 portion.

Nutrition Information...
Calories: 516   Protein: 13 g   Carbs: 62 g   Fat: 22 g

Cheddar Beef Quesadilla
Hot roast beef with all the toppings

Ingredients:
- 1 gluten free tortilla wrap
- 1 tsp. **margarine** or substitute
- 1 oz. (or 1/8 cup) meltable **soy cheese** or Cheddar cheese
- 2 oz. **roast beef deli meat**
- 1 thin slice onion
- 1 packet **horseradish sauce** (optional)

Stovetop Instructions:
Heat a skillet on medium heat. Lightly butter one side of a tortilla wrap and place the buttered side down on the skillet. Evenly spread the cheese, sliced meat, onion and sauce over half the tortilla – fold over the empty side. Continue cooking until the bottom of the tortilla starts to brown. Flip the tortilla over with a spatula and brown the other side. It is done when the filling is hot and the outside is golden brown. Makes 1 portion.

Microwave Instructions:
Thinly spread margarine or butter on the wrap and place butter side down on a paper towel. Layer the cheese, sliced meat, onion and sauce on the tortilla. Microwave on the paper towel on high power for 1 ½ to 2 minutes, or until the fillings are hot and the cheese melted. Allow to cool slightly, fold over in half, and cut into wedges. Makes 1 portion.

Nutrition Information...
Calories: 453   Protein: 19 g   Carbs: 33 g   Fat: 24 g

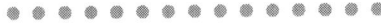

Crunchy Chicken Quesadilla
A surprise ingredient creates satisfying crunch

Ingredients:
- 1 gluten free tortilla wrap
- 1 tsp. **margarine** or substitute
- 1 oz. (or 1/8 cup) meltable **soy cheese** or dairy cheese
- 10 **corn chips**, broken up
- ½ -5 oz. can **cooked chicken**, drained (or 1/3 cup cooked chicken, diced)

Stovetop Instructions:
Heat a skillet on medium heat. Lightly butter one side of a tortilla wrap and place the buttered side down on the skillet. Evenly spread the cheese, corn chips, and chicken over half the tortilla – fold over the empty side. Continue cooking until the bottom of the tortilla starts to brown. Flip the tortilla over with a spatula and brown the other side. It is done when the filling is hot and the outside is golden brown. Makes 1 portion.

Microwave Instructions:
Thinly spread margarine or butter on the wrap and place butter side down on a paper towel. Layer the cheese, corn chips, and chicken on the tortilla. Microwave on the paper towel on high power for 1 ½ to 2 minutes, or until the fillings are hot and the cheese melted. Allow to cool slightly, fold over in half, and cut into wedges. Makes 1 portion.

Nutrition Information...
Calories: 527   Protein: 25 g   Carbs: 35 g   Fat: 30 g

Turkey, Bacon and Ranch Quesadilla
A classic sandwich combination in a wrap

Ingredients:
- 1 gluten free tortilla wrap
- 1 tsp. **margarine** or substitute
- 1 oz. (or 1/8 cup) meltable **soy cheese** or dairy cheese
- 2 oz. **deli turkey breast**
- 2 slices **bacon**, fully cooked
- 1 Tbsp. **Ranch dressing**

Stovetop Instructions:
Heat a skillet on medium heat. Lightly butter one side of a tortilla wrap and place the buttered side down on the skillet. Evenly spread the cheese, turkey, bacon and dressing over half the tortilla – fold over the empty side. Continue cooking until the bottom of the tortilla starts to brown. Flip the tortilla over with a spatula and brown the other side. It is done when the filling is hot and the outside is golden brown. Makes 1 portion.

Microwave Instructions:
Thinly spread margarine or butter on the wrap and place butter side down on a paper towel. Layer the cheese, turkey, bacon and dressing on the tortilla. Microwave on the paper towel on high power for 1 ½ to 2 minutes, or until the fillings are hot and the cheese melted. Allow to cool slightly, fold over in half, and cut into wedges. Makes 1 portion.

Nutrition Information...
Calories: 551   Protein: 23 g   Carbs: 33 g   Fat: 34 g

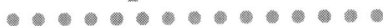

Smoked Sausage Quesadilla
Something different for lunch or dinner

Ingredients:
- ♦ 1 gluten free tortilla wrap
- ♦ 1 tsp. **margarine** or substitute
- ♦ 1 oz. (or 1/8 cup) meltable **soy cheese** or dairy cheese
- ♦ 1 serving **turkey smoked sausage**, cut into coins
- ♦ 6 slices pickle
- ♦ 1 tsp. **mustard**

Stovetop Instructions:
Heat a skillet on medium heat. Lightly butter one side of a tortilla wrap and place the buttered side down on the skillet. Evenly spread the cheese, sausage, pickle and mustard over half the tortilla – fold over the empty side. Continue cooking until the bottom of the tortilla starts to brown. Flip the tortilla over with a spatula and brown the other side. It is done when the filling is hot and the outside is golden brown. Makes 1 portion.

Microwave Instructions:
Thinly spread margarine or butter on the wrap and place butter side down on a paper towel. Layer the cheese, sausage, pickle and mustard on the tortilla. Microwave on the paper towel on high power for 1 ½ to 2 minutes, or until the fillings are hot and the cheese melted. Allow to cool slightly, fold over in half, and cut into wedges. Makes 1 portion.

Nutrition Information...
Calories: 461   Protein: 17 g   Carbs: 35 g   Fat: 27 g

Cream Cheese and Pineapple Quesadilla

A bit more like dessert than a meal

Ingredients:
- ◆ 1 gluten free tortilla wrap
- ◆ 1 tsp. **margarine** or substitute
- ◆ 1 oz. soy or dairy **cream cheese**
- ◆ 1 -4 oz. snack cup pineapple tidbits, drained
- ◆ 1 slice **turkey ham**, diced

Stovetop Instructions:
Heat a skillet on medium heat. Lightly butter one side of a tortilla wrap and place the buttered side down on the skillet. Evenly spread the cream cheese over half the tortilla and top with the well drained pineapple and ham – fold over the empty side. Continue cooking until the bottom of the tortilla starts to brown. Flip the tortilla over with a spatula and brown the other side. It is done when the filling is hot and the outside is golden brown. Makes 1 portion.

Microwave Instructions:
Thinly spread margarine or butter on the wrap and place butter side down on a paper towel. Spread the cream cheese over the tortilla and top with the well drained pineapple and ham. Microwave on the paper towel on high power for 1 ½ to 2 minutes, or until the fillings are hot and the cheese melted. Allow to cool slightly, fold over in half, and cut into wedges. Makes 1 portion.

Nutrition Information...
Calories: 425   Protein: 13 g   Carbs: 47 g   Fat: 22 g

Breakfast Quesadilla
Breakfast for a sleep-in day

Ingredients:
- ◆ 1 gluten free tortilla wrap
- ◆ 1 oz. **soy mozzarella cheese**, or dairy mozzarella
- ◆ 1 oz. **chorizo** sausage, or vegan **soy chorizo**, or **breakfast sausage**
- ◆ 2 large eggs, scrambled

Stovetop Instructions:
Heat a skillet on medium heat. Lightly butter one side of a tortilla wrap and place the buttered side down on the skillet. Evenly spread the cheese, sausage and cooked egg over half the tortilla – fold over the empty side. Continue cooking until the bottom of the tortilla starts to brown. Flip the tortilla over with a spatula and brown the other side. It is done when the filling is hot and the outside is golden brown. Makes 1 portion.

Microwave Instructions:
Thinly spread margarine or butter on the wrap and place butter side down on a paper towel. Layer the cheese, sausage and cooked egg on the tortilla. Microwave on the paper towel on high power for 1 ½ to 2 minutes, or until the fillings are hot and the cheese melted. Allow to cool slightly, fold over in half, and cut into wedges. Makes 1 portion.

Nutrition Information...
Calories: 522   Protein: 20 g   Carbs: 31 g   Fat: 34 g

*C*reative Cooking...
Add green chilies or salsa; sour cream; onions and peppers; or guacamole.

Tuna Melt Tostada

The classic open faced sandwich another way

Ingredients:

- ♦   1 tostada shell (100% corn)
- ♦   2 oz. tuna salad
- ♦   1 oz. **soy or dairy cheese**, shredded

Oven/Oven/Toaster Oven Directions:

Preheat the oven or toaster oven to Broil.

Spread the tostada with prepared tuna salad. Top with your choice of cheese. Place on an oven safe pan and put under the broiler. Watch carefully as this may burn if you go on an errand. The cheese should melt in 3 to 5 minutes. Makes 1 portion.

Nutrition Information...
Calories: 168   Protein: 12 g   Carbs: 15 g   Fat: 10 g

*S*hopping Tip...
Most corn tostadas and corn tortilla chips are gluten free. Check with the manufacturer if you are unsure. Always check *seasoned* corn chips as many have wheat as an ingredient.

If you can tolerate corn, tostadas are one of the most economical bread or cracker replacements. Often you can get 12-16 in a bag for less than $2. Thin and crunchy, they give needed texture to your gluten free diet.

Barbeque Chicken Tostada
Quick and tangy take on lunch

Ingredients:
- 1 tostada shell (100% corn)
- ½ -5 oz. can **cooked chicken**, drained (or 1/3 cup cooked chicken); or ¼ cup **seasoned tofu**
- 2 Tbsp. **barbeque sauce**
- 1 oz. **soy or dairy cheese**, shredded

Oven/Toaster Oven Directions:
Preheat the toaster oven to Broil.

Combine the drained, cooked chicken and barbeque sauce. Spread the chicken on the tostada. Top with your choice of cheese. Place on an oven safe pan and put under the broiler. Watch carefully as this may burn quickly. The cheese should melt in 3 to 5 minutes. Makes 1 portion.

Nutrition Information...
Calories: 307   Protein: 21 g   Carbs: 24 g   Fat: 11g

Philly Cheese Tostada

*If you have the time, sauté the onions
first for extra flavor*

Ingredients:
- 1 tostada shell (100% corn)
- 2 oz. **deli roast beef**
- 1 oz. white **soy** or **dairy Provolone cheese**
- 2 thin slices onion
- Several spicy pepper rings

Oven/Toaster Oven Directions:
Preheat the toaster oven to the highest heat setting and Broil. Layer the roast beef, onion and pepper rings on the tostada. Top with your choice of cheese. Place on an oven safe pan and put under the broiler. Watch carefully as this may burn quickly. The cheese should melt in 3 to 5 minutes. Makes 1 portion.

Nutrition Information...
Calories: 188   Protein: 18 g   Carbs: 10 g   Fat: 6 g

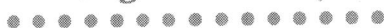

Pizza Tostada

*It doesn't get easier than this for a snack or lunch – you may
want to make multiples*

Ingredients:

- ♦ 1 tostada shell (100% corn)
- ♦ 2 Tbsp. **pizza sauce**
- ♦ 1 oz. **soy or dairy cheese**, shredded
- ♦ 6 slices **pepperoni** or vegan alternative
- ♦ 1/8 tsp. oregano

Oven/Toaster Oven Directions:

Preheat the toaster oven to Broil.
Top the tostada with pizza sauce. Layer on cheese, pepperoni (or
other toppings) and the oregano. Place on an oven safe pan and
put under the broiler. Watch carefully as this may burn quickly.
The cheese should melt in 3 to 5 minutes. Makes 1 portion.

Nutrition Information...
Calories: 184   Protein: 8 g   Carbs: 11 g   Fat: 10 g

Chili Cheese Tostada
Leftover chili makes an easy snack

Ingredients:
- ♦ 1 tostada shell (100% corn)
- ♦ 1/4 cup prepared **chili con carne,** or **vegetarian chili**
- ♦ 1 oz. **soy or dairy cheese,** shredded
- ♦ 1/8 tsp. **taco seasoning mix**

Oven/Toaster Oven Directions:
Preheat the toaster oven to Broil.
Top the tostada with chili. Add the cheese and taco seasoning. Place on an oven safe pan and put under the broiler. Watch carefully as this may burn. The cheese should melt in 3 to 5 minutes. Makes 1 portion.

Nutrition Information...
Calories: 174   Protein: 11 g   Carbs: 13 g   Fat: 7 g

*C*reative Cooking...
Add extra toppings - pepper rings, green chilies, minced fresh onion.
Any of the chili recipes in this book can be used for this recipe.

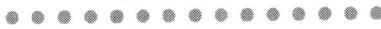

Tostada Marguerite
Fresh tomato pizza with basil

Ingredients:
- 1 tostada shell (100% corn)
- 2 Tbsp. **marinara sauce**
- 1 oz. **mozzarella soy** or dairy cheese, shredded
- 2-3 slices of ripe tomato
- 1/8 tsp. basil, dried, *or* 1 teaspoon fresh sliced basil

Oven/Toaster Oven Directions:
Preheat the toaster oven to Broil.
Top the tostada with the marinara sauce. Layer with the fresh tomato, cheese, and a sprinkle of basil. Place on an oven safe pan and put under the broiler. Watch carefully as this may burn quickly. The cheese should melt in 3 to 5 minutes. Makes 1 portion.

Nutrition Information...
Calories: 134   Protein: 6 g   Carbs: 11 g   Fat: 6 g

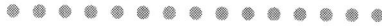

Chicky Tostada

Add fresh vegetables of choice like diced tomato, shredded carrot, and thin sliced bell pepper.

Ingredients:

- ♦ 1 tostada shell (100% corn)
- ♦ 2 Tbsp. **hummus**
- ♦ 1 oz. **soy or dairy cheese**, shredded

Oven/Toaster Oven Directions:

Preheat the toaster oven to Broil.

Spread the hummus on the tostada. Add any vegetables and top with your choice of cheese. Place on an oven safe pan and put under the broiler. Watch carefully as this may burn quickly. The cheese should melt in 3 to 5 minutes. Makes 1 portion.

Nutrition Information...

Calories: 156   Protein: 7 g   Carbs: 11 g   Fat: 8 g

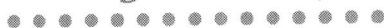

Chicken Curry Tostada
A hint of curry brightens chicken salad

Ingredients:
- ♦ 1 tostada shell (100% corn)
- ♦ ½- 5 oz. can **cooked chicken**, drained (or 1/3 cup cooked chicken); or ¼ cup **seasoned tofu**
- ♦ 1 small stalk celery, thinly sliced
- ♦ 1 Tbsp. **mayonnaise**
- ♦ 1 Tbsp. golden raisins
- ♦ 1/4 tsp. **curry powder**
- ♦ 1 oz. **soy or dairy cheese**, shredded

Oven/Toaster Oven Directions:
Preheat the toaster oven to Broil.
Combine the well-drained, cooked chicken with the mayonnaise, chopped celery, raisins, and curry powder. Top the tostada and add a layer of cheese. Place on an oven safe pan and put under the broiler. Watch carefully as this may burn. The cheese should melt in 3 to 5 minutes. Makes 1 portion.

Nutrition Information...
Calories: 311   Protein: 21 g   Carbs: 17 g   Fat: 15 g

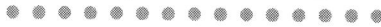

Refried Bean Tostada
Lower fat snack high in protein

Ingredients:
- ♦ 1 tostada shell (100% corn)
- ♦ 2 Tbsp. **refried beans**
- ♦ 2 Tbsp. salsa
- ♦ 1 oz. **soy or dairy cheese**, shredded

Oven/Toaster Oven Directions:
Preheat the oven or toaster oven to Broil.
Top the tostada with the refried beans, salsa and layer of cheese. Place on an oven safe pan and put under the broiler. Watch carefully. The cheese should melt in 3 to 5 minutes. Makes 1 portion.

Nutrition Information...
Calories: 148   Protein: 7 g   Carbs: 14 g   Fat: 5 g

BLT Tostada
A traditional combination on a crispy base

Ingredients:
- 1 tostada shell (100% corn)
- 2 slices fully cooked **bacon**
- 1 oz. **soy or dairy cheese**, shredded
- 1 slice tomato
- 1/4 cup shredded lettuce
- 2 tsp. **Ranch salad dressing**

Oven/Toaster Oven Directions:
Preheat the oven or toaster oven to Broil.

Top the tostada with the cooked bacon slices, the diced tomato, and the cheese. Place on an oven safe pan and put under the broiler. Watch carefully. The cheese should melt in 3 to 5 minutes. Top with lettuce and a drizzle of Ranch dressing. Makes 1 portion.

Nutrition Information...
Calories: 221   Protein: 10 g   Carbs: 9 g   Fat: 14 g

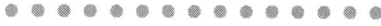

Turkey & Cranberry Tostada
Crisp, crunchy, and slightly sweet – a great combination

Ingredients:
- ♦ 1 tostada shell (100% corn)
- ♦ 2 oz. **deli turkey breast**
- ♦ 1 strip celery, sliced thin
- ♦ 1 Tbsp. dried cranberries
- ♦ 1 oz. **soy or dairy cheese**, shredded

Oven/Toaster Oven Directions:
Preheat the oven or toaster oven to Broil.

Top the tostada with the sliced turkey. Top with the celery, cranberries and cheese. Place on an oven safe pan and put under the broiler. Watch carefully as this may burn quickly. The cheese should melt in 3 to 5 minutes. Makes 1 portion.

Nutrition Information...
Calories: 194   Protein: 16 g   Carbs: 16 g   Fat: 5 g

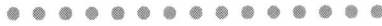

Health Crunch Tostada
Crunchy and good

Ingredients:
- ♦ 1 tostada shell (100% corn)
- ♦ 2 Tbsp. **hummus**
- ♦ 1 tsp. sunflower seeds
- ♦ 1 tsp. walnut pieces
- ♦ 2 Tbsp. diced fresh apple
- ♦ 2 Tbsp. carrot, shredded
- ♦ 1 tsp. tahini or **salad dressing**
- ♦ 1 oz. **soy or dairy cheese**, shredded (optional)

Oven/Toaster Oven Directions:
Preheat the oven or toaster oven to Broil.

Spread the hummus on the tostada. Layer with the nuts, apples, and carrot. Drizzle with the tahini. Top with cheese if desired. Place on an oven safe pan and put under the broiler. Watch carefully as this may burn quickly. The cheese should melt in 3 to 5 minutes. Makes 1 portion.

Nutrition Information...
Calories: 406   Protein: 13 g   Carbs: 19 g   Fat: 31 g

Ham & Cheese Tostada
Try different cheeses and mustards for variety

Ingredients:
- 1 tostada shell (100% corn)
- 1 tsp. **Dijon mustard**
- 2 1/2 oz. **deli ham**
- 1 oz. **soy or dairy cheese**, shredded

Oven/Toaster Oven Directions:
Preheat the oven or toaster oven to Broil.

Spread the mustard on the tostada. Top with the ham and cheese. Place on an oven safe pan and put under the broiler. Watch carefully as this may burn if you go on an errand. The cheese should melt in 3 to 5 minutes. Makes 1 portion.

Nutrition Information...
Calories: 215   Protein: 17 g   Carbs: 10 g   Fat: 12 g

Thai Chicken Tostada

Wake up your day with something different

Ingredients:

♦   1 tostada shell (100% corn)
♦   ½- 5 oz. can **cooked chicken**, drained (or 1/3 cup cooked chicken); or ¼ cup **seasoned tofu**
♦   1/2 tsp. **soy sauce or tamari**
♦   Juice of ¼ lime
♦   1/4 tsp. toasted sesame oil
♦   2 Tbsp. bean or broccoli sprouts
♦   1 oz. **soy or dairy cheese**, shredded

Oven/Toaster Oven Directions:

Preheat the oven or toaster oven to Broil.

Combine the chicken, soy sauce, lime juice and sesame oil. Layer with the sprouts and top with the cheese. Place on an oven safe pan and put under the broiler. Watch carefully as this may burn quickly. The cheese should melt in 3 to 5 minutes. Makes 1 portion.

Nutrition Information...
Calories: 256   Protein: 22 g   Carbs: 10 g   Fat: 12 g

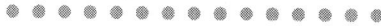

Greek Tostada
Greek flavors make a great snack

Ingredients:

- ♦ 1 tostada shell (100% corn)
- ♦ ½ -5 oz. can **cooked chicken**, drained (or 1/3 cup cooked chicken); or ¼ cup. **seasoned tofu**
- ♦ 1 slice tomato, diced
- ♦ 2 Tbsp. feta cheese, crumbled; or dairy free cheese
- ♦ 1/8 tsp. oregano, dried

Oven/Toaster Oven Directions:
Preheat the oven or toaster oven to Broil.

Layer the chicken, tomato, cheese and oregano on the tostada. Place on an oven safe pan and put under the broiler. Watch carefully as this may burn quickly. The cheese should melt in 3 to 5 minutes. Makes 1 portion.

Nutrition Information...
Calories: 217   Protein: 18 g   Carbs: 8 g   Fat: 11 g

Pizza

A pie a day keeps the blues at bay

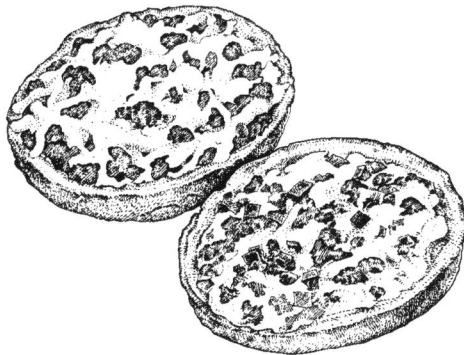

Probably the most popular food at college and beyond is the pizza. If you're gluten free, you can expect to pay big bucks for a gluten free crust or restaurant GF pizza. Here to the rescue are some recipes designed for dorm or apartment living without the expense of packaged crusts, or purchasing a shelf full of gluten free specialty flours. These tasty recipes will "kill the crave" for pizza when that smell wafts down the hall from another dorm room.

For those of you who may have the kitchen facilities and the interest to bake up some shells, there is a simple pizza crust recipe ready to try. I debated on putting a pizza crust in this book because of the baking skill and equipment required, and then I happened on this recipe by accident doing another cooking test. The crust does not need yeast or a big mixer, and makes a crisp, hold-it-in-your-hand thin crust. Further more, you can make a big bag of pizza crust mix and make it up one crust at a time. Make several at a time and you can freeze a couple for quick meals in the future.

Finishing the topped pizza on a very high heat – broil or 450°F. or more – will give the pizza a wood fired pizza look and taste. Be careful not to forget about your pizza when using higher heats because it will burn if not watched. The improvement in taste is worth the extra effort.

On the creative front, pizza can be made on gluten free buns, English muffins, bagels, polenta, or corn tostadas. Whatever you have, with whatever toppings you can find, will help fill your pizza appetite.

Note: Items listed in **bold** in the recipes have a higher incidence of containing gluten – it's a *reminder* to always check the label or directly with the manufacturer.

• • • • • • • • • • • • • • • •

Simple Crispy Pizza Crust

Gluten free, casein free, yeast free, egg free

Ingredients:

- ♦ 1 cup gluten free flour mix (purchased, or 1 cup rice flour, 2/3 c. potato starch, 1/3 c. tapioca starch mixed together – just use one cup of the mix)
- ♦ 1 tsp. **baking powder**
- ♦ 1 tsp. Xanthan gum
- ♦ 1/4 tsp. baking soda
- ♦ 1/4 tsp. salt
- ♦ 1/4 tsp. oregano
- ♦ 1/8 tsp. garlic powder
- ♦ 1 1/2 Tbsp. vegetable or olive oil
- ♦ 1/2 cup **rice, soy, almond, or dairy milk**

This recipe makes one 12" crust or 2- 6" individual crusts depending on how you form the dough.

Preheat oven to 375° F. Combine the dry ingredients in a mixing bowl. Add the milk and oil. Mix well for 1 minute. The dough will collect into a ball as you stir. Turn out the dough onto a non-stick baking pan. Place a piece of plastic wrap over the dough. With your hand and fingers, press the dough out evenly into a round (or other shape). Remove the plastic wrap. Cooking note: The thinner the crust, the crispier it will be. It will rise in the oven to about double the thickness as the raw crust.

Place into the oven and bake for about 10 minutes, until light brown. Remove from the oven and 1.) Sauce, add toppings, and broil for 8-10 minutes more; OR, 2.) Cool the pizza crust to room temperature, wrap well and freeze or refrigerate for future use.

Nutrition Information for one 6" crust...
Calories: 387   Protein: 3 g   Carbs: 75 g   Fat: 8 g

Bulk Pizza Crust Mix

*Make a big batch and dip into it to make one crust at a time...
just mix and bake*

Ingredients:

- ♦ 6 cups gluten free flour mix (purchased; or 3 c. rice flour, 2 c. potato starch, 1 c. tapioca starch mixed together)
- ♦ 2 Tbsp. baking powder
- ♦ 2 Tbsp. Xanthan gum
- ♦ 1 1/2 tsp. baking soda
- ♦ 1 1/2 tsp. oregano
- ♦ 1 tsp. salt
- ♦ 3/4 tsp. garlic powder

A bulk mix can save time in the kitchen. It is important to store this in an air tight container or zip bag. Use within 1 month. Combine all the ingredients, **mixing very well before every use**. Makes about 12 individual 6" crusts when prepared as below.

To use:

This recipe will make one 6" individual crust. Preheat oven to 375°F. Measure out a level 1/2 cup of the mix into a small mixing bowl. Add 1/4 cup milk and 3/4 tablespoon vegetable oil. Mix well with a spoon for 1 minute. Turn out the dough onto a non-stick baking pan. Place a piece of plastic wrap over the dough. With your hand and fingers, press the dough out into a round (or other shape). Remove the plastic wrap. Cooking Note: The thinner the crust, the crispier it will be. It will rise in the oven to about double the thickness as the raw crust.

Place into the oven and bake for about 10 minutes. Remove from the oven and sauce, add the toppings, and turn the oven to *broil* for 8-10 minutes more.

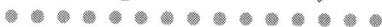

Dairy Free, Gluten Free Cheese Pizza

Getting soy cheese to melt can be a challenge. It has to reach a very hot temperature to act and look like dairy cheese. See how it's done below.

Ingredients:

- ♦ 1 -6" GF par-baked pizza crust, purchased or from the recipe on page 155
- ♦ 2 Tbsp. **pizza sauce, purchased** or from recipe on the next page
- ♦ 1 oz. **soy mozzarella cheese**, or dairy mozzarella cheese, shredded or diced
- ♦ dash oregano

Preheat the oven or toaster oven to Broil.

(If you are using the pizza crust recipe on page 149, bake the crust at 375 F. and after removing it from the oven, turn the oven or toaster oven to *broil* while you add your toppings.)

Top the crust with the pizza sauce spreading to the edges. Crumble the soy cheese over the crust and sprinkle lightly with oregano. Put into the oven for 7-10 minutes, or until the cheese has melted and the edges are lightly browned. Watch carefully as food tends to burn under such high heat.

Nutrition Information...
Calories: 389   Protein: 4 g   Carbs: 58 g   Fat: 14 g

Suggested pans for use under the broiler:

The oven broiler emits such high heat that many thin metal baking pans will buckle permanently. Instead, use a heavier metal baking tray, the toaster oven baking tray, oven proof glass pie plates, or aluminum pie plates. Check the bottom of silicone bake ware for the maximum temperature before using under the broiler.

Quick Pizza Sauce

A spicy, slightly sweet sauce made in a minute

Ingredients:

- 1 -8 oz. can **tomato sauce**
- 1 Tbsp. onion flakes, dehydrated
- 1 Tbsp. **soy Parmesan cheese**, or dairy Parmesan
- 1 tsp. olive oil
- 1/2 tsp. basil
- 1/2 tsp. oregano
- 1/4 tsp. garlic powder
- 1 packet sugar (optional)

Recipes Instructions:

Combine all ingredients in a covered and vented 2-cup microwave safe container. Heat and stir in 30 second intervals until hot. Makes enough for four 6" inch pizzas. Can be cooled and refrigerated for up to 1 week.

Nutrition Information...
Calories: 58   Protein: 2 g   Carbs: 10 g   Fat: 1 g

Cooking Tip:

The sauce does not need to be hot to go on pizza. Cooking it blends the flavors of the ingredients. If you do not have a microwave, you can just combine the ingredients and use.

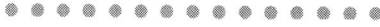

Breakfast Pizza
What a way to start the day

Ingredients:
- ♦ 1 - 6" GF par-baked pizza crust, purchased or from the recipe on page 155
- ♦ 1 Tbsp. **non-dairy or dairy cream cheese**
- ♦ 1 large egg, scrambled
- ♦ ½ oz. **shredded soy mozzarella cheese**, or dairy mozzarella

Preheat the oven to *broil*. Place a pizza crust on a broiler safe pan. Top the pizza crust with the cream cheese, spreading to the edges. Cook the scrambled egg and crumble that over the top. Finish off with the cheese. Put into the oven for 7-10 minutes, or until the cheese has melted.

Nutrition Information...
Calories: 443   Protein: 8 g   Carbs: 58 g   Fat: 18 g

Scrambling an egg in the microwave...
Break an egg into a microwave safe container or mug. Add 1 teaspoon milk or water and beat with a fork. Cook covered on high for 1 minute, then stir from the sides and bottom with a spoon. Continue to cook and stir in 20 second intervals until the egg is just firm. It will cook more upon standing.

Creative Cooking...
Add crumbled breakfast sausage, soy chorizo sausage, or diced tomatoes or peppers on the layer under the cheese.

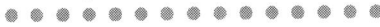

Peanut Butter and Jelly Pizza
Quick and simple to make, a great breakfast or snack

Ingredients:
- ♦ 1 - 6" GF par-baked pizza crust, purchased or from the recipe on page 155
- ♦ 1-2 Tbsp. peanut butter, or nut butter
- ♦ 1 Tbsp. jelly
- ♦ 10 miniature **marshmallows**

Recipe Instructions:
Preheat the oven to 425° F.

Top the crust with the peanut butter, spreading it to the edges. Drizzle the jelly over the top and dot the pizza with mini marshmallows. Put into the oven for 8-10 minutes, or until the marshmallows have melted and are lightly brown. Check often so that it doesn't burn. Allow to cool slightly – this will give new meaning to pizza mouth if you try to eat it too soon!

Nutrition Information...
Calories: 623   Protein: 11 g   Carbs: 85 g   Fat: 26 g

Extra Cheesy Pizza
Three cheeses for fun

Ingredients:
- ♦ 1 - 6" GF par-baked pizza crust, purchased or from the recipe on page 155
- ♦ 1 Tbsp. **non-dairy or dairy cream cheese**
- ♦ 1 Tbsp. **soy Parmesan cheese**, or dairy Parmesan
- ♦ Dash oregano, basil, or crushed red pepper
- ♦ 1 oz. **mozzarella style soy cheese**, or dairy mozzarella cheese

Recipe Instructions:
Preheat the oven to *broil*.

Top the crust with the cream cheese, spreading it to the edges. Top with the Parmesan cheese and spices. Crumble the soy cheese over the crust. Put into the oven for 8-10 minutes, or until the cheese has melted and is lightly browned. Check often so that it doesn't burn.

Nutrition Information...
Calories: 472   Protein: 9 g   Carbs: 59 g   Fat: 21 g

Athena's Pizza

Greek pizza tasty enough for the gods

Ingredients:
- 1 - 6" GF par-baked pizza crust, purchased or from the recipe on page 155
- 1/2 tsp. olive oil
- 1/8 tsp. garlic powder
- 1/4 cup tomato, diced
- 3 Tbsp. crumbled Feta cheese; or meltable white **soy cheese**
- 6 kalamata olives, pitted, cut in half
- 1/8 tsp. oregano, dried

Recipe Instructions:
Preheat the oven to *broil*.

Rub the crust with the olive oil. Sprinkle with garlic powder, and then evenly spread on the diced tomatoes. Crumble the cheese over the tomatoes. Cut the olives in half and place on top. Shake on a little oregano to taste. Put into the oven for 8-10 minutes, or until the cheese has melted and is lightly browned. Check often so that it doesn't burn.

Nutrition Information...
Calories: 462   Protein: 6 g   Carbs: 60 g   Fat: 22 g

Spicy Shrimp Pizza
A special pizza for academic milestones

Ingredients:
- 1 - 6" GF par-baked pizza crust, purchased or from the recipe on page 155
- 1 Tbsp. **Ranch salad dressing**
- 2 oz. **shrimp**, canned, well drained (about ½ the can)
- 1 Tbsp. **barbeque sauce**
- 1 oz. **shredded mozzarella** soy cheese, or dairy mozzarella
- Sprinkle of dried red pepper flakes (optional)

Recipe Instructions:
Preheat the oven to *broil*.

Top the crust with the ranch dressing, spreading it to the edges. Spread the shrimp over the crust and drizzle with barbeque sauce. Top with cheese and red pepper (if desired). Put into the oven for 8-10 minutes, or until the cheese has melted and is lightly browned. Check often so that it doesn't burn.

Nutrition Information...
Calories: 602   Protein: 14 g   Carbs: 60 g   Fat: 32 g

Creative Cooking...
What to do with leftover shrimp? Make a quick shrimp salad with mayonnaise; garnish a salad; top almost any rice for the last few minutes of cooking; or toss with cooked garlic butter pasta.

Ham and Pineapple Pizza
Change up your pizza pattern

Ingredients:
- ♦ 1 - 6" GF par-baked pizza crust, purchased or from the recipe on page 155
- ♦ 1 Tbsp. **non-dairy or dairy cream cheese**
- ♦ 1 oz. **turkey ham**, diced or sliced
- ♦ 1 - 4 oz. snack pack pineapple tidbits, *well drained*
- ♦ 1 slice **soy cheese**, mozzarella, sliced

Recipe Instructions:
Preheat the oven to *broil*.

Top the crust with cream cheese, spreading it to the edges. For the next layer, add the diced ham and then the cheese. Drain the pineapple very well and spread over the crust. Put into the oven for 8-10 minutes, or until the cheese has melted and the pineapple is lightly browned. Check often so that it doesn't burn.

Nutrition Information...
Calories: 539   Protein: 11 g   Carbs: 76 g   Fat: 21 g

Crabmeat Salad Pizza
Very decadent – like hot crab dip on a crisp crust

Ingredients:
- ♦ 1 - 6" GF par-baked pizza crust, purchased or from the recipe on page 155
- ♦ 2 oz. **canned crab**, well drained (about ½ the can)
- ♦ 2 Tbsp. **mayonnaise**
- ♦ 1/8 tsp. **chili powder**
- ♦ 1 oz. **shredded mozzarella soy cheese**, or dairy mozzarella

Recipe Instructions:
Preheat the oven to *broil*.

Combine the drained crab, mayonnaise, and chili power. Spread onto the pizza crust. Top with cheese. Put into the oven for 8-10 minutes, or until the cheese has melted and is lightly browned. Check often so that it doesn't burn.

Nutrition Information...
Calories: 528   Protein: 10 g   Carbs: 59 g   Fat: 26 g

Creative Cooking...
What to do with leftover crab? Add it to Alfredo style pasta; mix it in to steamed rice and vegetables; or make crab salad with celery, onion, and salad dressing for a lunch sandwich filling.

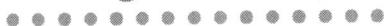

Refried Pizza
Mexican flavors make this pizza pop

Ingredients:
- 1 - 6" GF par-baked pizza crust, purchased or from the recipe on page 155
- 2 Tbsp. **refried beans, or bean dip**
- 1 oz. **shredded mozzarella soy cheese**, or dairy mozzarella
- 2 Tbsp. salsa
- 1/3 avocado, sliced

Recipe Instructions:
Preheat the oven to *broil*.

Top the crust with the refried beans, spreading it to the edges. Add a layer of salsa and then the cheese on top. Put into the oven for 8-10 minutes, or until the cheese has melted and is lightly browned. Check often so that it doesn't burn. Top with salsa and avocado slices.

Nutrition Information...
Calories: 547   Protein: 8 g   Carbs: 70 g   Fat: 25 g

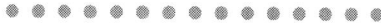
Reuben Pizza
Add some sauerkraut if you enjoy it

Ingredients:
- 1 - 6" GF par-baked pizza crust, purchased or from the recipe on page 155
- 1 Tbsp. **1000 Island**, or **Russian salad dressing**
- 2 oz. **deli cooked corned beef**, cut into small pieces
- 1 oz. white **soy cheese**, or dairy Swiss cheese

Recipe Instructions:
Preheat the oven to *broil*.

Top the crust with the 1000 Island or Russian dressing, spreading it to the edges. Cut the deli corned beef into strips and spread evenly across the crust. Top with the cheese. Put into the oven for 8-10 minutes, or until the cheese has melted and is lightly browned. Check often so that it doesn't burn.

Nutrition Information...
Calories: 576   Protein: 22 g   Carbs: 58 g   Fat: 28 g

Barbeque Pork Pizza

The open faced sandwich of the year for pork lovers

Ingredients:

- ♦ 1 - 6" GF par-baked pizza crust, purchased or from the recipe on page 155
- ♦ 2 oz. prepared **barbeque pork**
- ♦ 1 oz. shredded mozzarella **soy cheese**, or dairy mozzarella

Recipe Instructions:

Preheat the oven to *broil*.

Top the crust with the barbeque pork, spreading it to the edges. Top with the cheese. Put into the oven for 8-10 minutes, or until the cheese has melted and is lightly browned. Check often so that it doesn't burn.

Nutrition Information...
Calories: 502   Protein: 14 g   Carbs: 60 g   Fat: 21 g

*S*hopping Tip...
Barbeque pork can be purchased (check the ingredients) or made from leftover pork chops or roast. Some deli's carry a pork loin for slicing. Just cube the cooked pork and moisten with a GF barbeque sauce. Also good hot on a bun or English muffin.

Hummus Garden Pizza

*Flavorful chick pea spread topped off with melty cheese
and a garden of vegetables*

Ingredients:

- 1 - 6" GF par-baked pizza crust, purchased or from the recipe on page 155
- 2 Tbsp. **roasted garlic hummus**
- 1/3 carrot, shredded
- 1 Tbsp. red pepper, diced
- 1 oz. shredded mozzarella **soy cheese**, or dairy mozzarella
- 2 thin-slices fresh tomato

Recipe Instructions:

Preheat the oven to *broil*.

Top the crust with the hummus, spreading it to the edges. Add a layer of shredded carrot, diced red pepper, and then the cheese on top. Put into the oven for 8-10 minutes, or until the cheese has melted and is lightly browned. Check often so that it doesn't burn. Top with tomato slices.

Nutrition Information...
Calories: 451   Protein: 6 g   Carbs: 65 g   Fat: 18 g

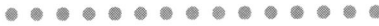

Bruschetta Pizza

*Purchased bruschetta spread uplifts this pizza
to gourmet status*

Ingredients:

- ♦ 1 - 6" GF par-baked pizza crust, purchased or from the recipe on page 155
- ♦ 1/4 cup **bruschetta spread**
- ♦ 1 oz. shredded mozzarella **soy cheese**, or dairy mozzarella
- ♦ 4 black olives, sliced

Recipe Instructions:

Preheat the oven to *broil*.

Top the crust with the bruschetta spread to the edges. Add the cheese and dot with the black olives. Put into the oven for 8-12 minutes, or until the cheese has melted and is lightly browned. Check often so that it doesn't burn.

Nutrition Information...
Calories: 564   Protein: 7 g   Carbs: 63 g   Fat: 30 g

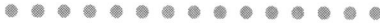

Meat Lovers Pizza Poppers
Add more meats if you have them

Ingredients:
- ♦ 1 GF hamburger bun, split
- ♦ 2 Tbsp. **pizza sauce**
- ♦ 1/2 oz. **pepperoni**
- ♦ 1 tsp. **bacon bits**
- ♦ 1 tsp. **Parmesan cheese**
- ♦ 1/2 oz. mozzarella **soy cheese**; or dairy mozzarella

Recipe Directions:
Split the hamburger roll and put on a toaster oven tray. Spread the pizza sauce evenly over the halves. Sprinkle the bacon bits, Parmesan cheese and mozzarella evenly over each half. Top with the pepperoni. Broil in a toaster oven or standard oven for 8-12 minutes until the cheese is melted. Watch carefully.

Nutrition Information...
Calories: 402   Protein: 9 g   Carbs: 39 g   Fat: 22 g

Barbeque Chicken Pizza Poppers
Makes a great forth meal

Ingredients:
- 1 GF hamburger bun, split
- 1/4 cup **cooked chicken**, diced small
- 2 Tbsp. **barbeque sauce**
- 1/2 oz. mozzarella **soy cheese**; or dairy mozzarella cheese
- 1/4 tsp. oregano

Oven/Toaster Oven Directions:
Preheat the oven/toaster oven to 450° F.
Split the hamburger roll and put on a toaster oven tray.
Combine the cooked chicken meat and barbeque sauce in a
small bowl. Spread evenly over the roll halves. Sprinkle evenly
with the mozzarella and oregano. Bake for 8-12 minutes until
the cheese is melted.

Nutrition Information...
Calories: 396   Protein: 15 g   Carbs: 46 g   Fat: 16g

*C*reative Cooking...
Add sliced green or red onion, diced red or green pepper, or
bacon bits under the cheese.

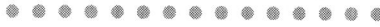

Ranch Bagel Pizza
A favorite combination of tastes

Ingredients:
- 1 large GF bagel
- 2 Tbsp. **Ranch dressing**
- 1/2 oz. mozzarella **soy cheese**; or dairy mozzarella cheese
- 1/4 tsp. oregano
- 1/4 oz. **pepperoni** (about 8 slices) or vegan alternative

Oven/Toaster Oven Directions:
Preheat the oven/toaster oven to 425° F.
Spread each half of the bagel with Ranch dressing. Evenly spread the mozzarella cheese over each and sprinkle with oregano. Top with the pepperoni.

Bake for 10-15 minutes, or until the cheese is melted.

Nutrition Information...
Calories: 595   Protein: 18 g Carbs: 72 g   Fat: 25 g

*V*egan Friendly...
Instead of pepperoni, add crumbled seasoned tofu or soy chorizo, or just add a garden of vegetables like broccoli, shredded carrot, or diced green and red peppers under the cheese.

Garlic Chicken Bagel Pizza
Makes a delicious lunch on the quick

Ingredients:
- 1 large GF bagel
- 1 Tbsp. **mayonnaise**
- 1 tsp. soy **Parmesan cheese**; or dairy Parmesan cheese
- 1/4 tsp. garlic powder
- 1/4 cup **cooked chicken**, diced
- 1 oz. mozzarella **soy cheese**; or dairy mozzarella cheese
- 1/4 tsp. oregano

Oven/Toaster Oven Directions:
Preheat the oven/toaster oven to 425° F.
Spread each half of the bagel with half the mayonnaise and then shake the Parmesan cheese over the two halves and a sprinkle of garlic powder. Top with the cooked chicken meat and then the mozzarella cheese. Dust the oregano on top.

Bake for 10-15 minutes, or until the cheese is melted.

Nutrition Information...
Calories: 625   Protein: 30 g   Carbs: 72 g   Fat: 23 g

S hopping Tip...
There are several brands of gluten free canned chicken meat that may be helpful to you. It's convenient for the dorm kitchen being already cooked −just drain and flake for pizza, casseroles, or salad.

Noodles and Pasta

When nothing but a Carb Blast will do

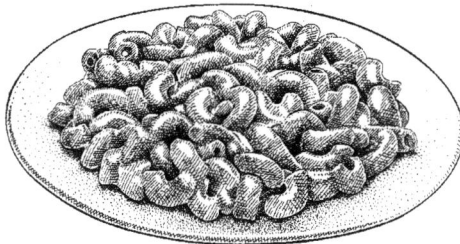

Pasta Cooking

Microwave Instructions. To cook plain pasta in a microwave, use a microwave safe container of *at least* a 2-quart size. Use 2/3 cup dry pasta for each serving. Don't try to cook more than 2-3 portions at a time in a 2-quart container.

Fill the container half full of water and microwave on full power for 5 minutes. Add the pasta and stir. Cook for 6 minutes on high and stir the pasta. Continue to cook and stir in 1-minute intervals for about 4 minutes more, depending on your microwave. Pasta should still be firm but tender. Let the pasta sit in the hot water for 2-4 minutes more to finish cooking. Pour the pasta into a colander in a sink to drain, being careful with the very hot water. You can rinse the pasta to remove extra starch or use it as it is.

Rice Cooker Instructions. Fill the rice cooker half-full of water and turn on. Wait until the water bubbles (boils), and add the pasta. Use 2/3 cup dry pasta for each serving. Don't try to cook more than 4 portions in a 3-cup rice cooker. Cook for about 6 minutes, stirring once. Turn the rice cooker to warm and cover. Wait for 5-8 minutes for the pasta to finish cooking in the hot water. Pour into a colander in a sink, being careful with the very hot water. You can rinse the pasta to remove extra starch or use it as it is.

Stovetop Instructions. Fill a 2 quart sauce pan 2/3 full of water. Place on stove and turn on to medium high heat. Wait until the water bubbles (boils), and add the pasta. Use 2/3 cup dry pasta for each serving. Cook for about 6 minutes, stirring once. Turn the heat off and cover. Wait for 5-8 minutes for the pasta to finish cooking in the hot water. Pour into a colander in a sink, being careful with the very hot water. You can rinse the pasta to remove extra starch or use it as it is.

Cooking Rice Pasta in One Pot.

Many of the pasta recipes in this book use a method of cooking pasta right in the sauce rather than in boiling water. While not a traditional method, this does work very well for dorm and apartment cooking. After many rounds of cooking trials, the brown rice pastas were found to cook nicely in many different types of sauces. For the ultimate convenience and safety of cooking in limited kitchen facilities, this is a great way to put some food on the table quickly.

When the recipe instructs you to put all the ingredients into the pot, it means the uncooked (or DRY) pasta too. The recipes are written with additional moisture so that the pasta absorbs the liquid and leaves a nice creamy sauce. The added starch from the pasta serves as a thickener. You also get all the nutrition from the pasta – nothing gets washed down the drain.

Thicker pasta sauces like a chunky vegetable sauce may need 1-2 Tablespoons extra water. You can always add more liquid near the end of cooking if it looks too dry - but you can't take it away - so you may want to wait until the end to judge.

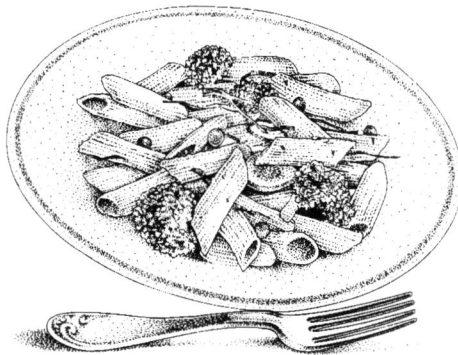

Cooking Rice Noodles

Rice noodles, or rice sticks as they are called in Asian grocery stores, are easy to prepare for snacks or meals. They are available in many widths and can easily become the gluten free college students "ramen noodles." One package generally makes 4 portions. Note: if you are very sensitive to gluten, you should trust only to rice noodles made in a dedicated gluten free facility.

Microwave Instructions.

The noodles usually only have to be soaked in hot water before they are ready to use. You don't need to cook them like pasta. Use 2 oz. (or ¼ of a block) for each serving. Don't try to cook more than 4 portions at a time in a 2 quart container. The noodles can be broken up at this point if you want shorter lengths. To prepare the rice noodles in a microwave, use a microwave safe container of at least a 2-quart size. Fill it half full of water and microwave on full power for 4 minutes. Add the noodles and stir.

Cook for 3-4 minutes on high and stir. Let the noodles sit in the hot water for 2-4 minutes more to finish cooking. Pour the noodles into a colander in a sink to drain, being careful with the hot water. Once drained, you can add an oriental sauce and vegetables, and microwave for 2-3 minutes more for a full meal or snack.

Rice Cooker Instructions.

Use 2 oz. (or ¼ of a block) dry rice noodles for each serving. Don't try to cook more than 4 portions at a time in a small rice cooker. Fill the rice cooker half-full of water and turn on. Wait until the water bubbles (boils), and add the noodles. The noodles can be broken up at this point if you want shorter lengths. Add the noodles and stir.

Cook for about 2-3 minutes, stirring once. Turn the rice cooker to the warm setting and cover. Wait 5-8 minutes for the noodles to finish cooking in the hot water. Pour into a colander in a sink, being careful with the hot water.

Gluten Free College Student Cookbook

Cooking Rice Noodles, continued

Stovetop Instructions.

Use 2 oz. (or ¼ of a block) for each serving. Don't try to cook more than 4 portions at a time in a small saucepan. Fill a 2 quart sauce pan 2/3 full of water. Place pan on stove and turn on to medium high heat. Wait until the water bubbles (boils). The noodles can be broken up at this point if you want shorter lengths. Add the noodles and stir.

Cook for about 2-3 minutes, stirring once. Turn the stove off and cover. Wait for 5-8 minutes for the noodles to finish cooking in the hot water. Pour into a colander in a sink, being careful with the hot water.

Please note: all microwaves and all stoves cook at a different rate. The timing in the instructions is a **guideline**. *It may take less or more time in your appliance.*

Creative Cooking...

Use rice sticks in the recipes or develop your own noodle creations. The noodles can be used as you would spaghetti, or in stir fry's. Break the dry sticks into hot, simmering broth for a quick noodle soup. Cooked noodles can also be drizzled with a vinaigrette style salad dressing for a cold noodle salad with vegetables.

You will soon find that the possibilities are endless!

Note: Items listed in **bold** in the recipes have a higher incidence of containing gluten – it's a **reminder** to always check the label or directly with the manufacturer.

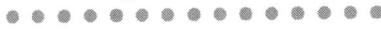

GF/CF Macaroni and Cheese

A one-pot recipe for creamy, cheesy macaroni and cheese. No boiling water, straining pasta, or working hard to make a quick meal or snack.

Ingredients:

- ◆ 2 oz. brown rice pasta (about 2/3 cup dry pasta)
- ◆ 3/4 cup **chicken stock** (*OR* one chicken/vegetable **bouillon cube** and 3/4 cup water)
- ◆ 3/4 cup **rice, soy or almond milk**
- ◆ 2 oz. *meltable* **soy cheese**
- ◆ 1 tsp. **Worcestershire sauce** (optional)
- ◆ 1/4 tsp. **mustard powder** (optional)

Rice Cooker Directions:

Put all ingredients into rice cooker. Turn on, cover and stir once in a while. When pasta is almost cooked, about 12 minutes, turn the cooker to warm. Allow the pasta to finish cooking for about 5 minutes. Makes 2 portions.

Microwave Directions:

In a 2 quart microwavable container, combine pasta, stock and milk. Cook for 8 minutes. Stir, and add cheese and seasonings. Continue cooking for 30 second intervals until cheese is melted. Let sit for 5 minutes. Stir and serve.

Nutrition Information...
Calories 267   Protein: 7 g   Carbs: 34 g   Fat: 10 g

*S*hopping Tip... This recipe works well for brown rice and quinoa pasta, but not for corn or artichoke pasta.

C reative Cooking for Macaroni and Cheese...

♦ **Add** steamed vegetables (like broccoli, carrots, red and green peppers) for Pasta Primavera. If you are using a rice cooker, the vegetables can cook in the steamer basket as you are cooking the pasta

♦ **Add** diced bacon, ham, or pepperoni at the end of cooking. A meat lover's delight.

♦ **Add** a large spoonful of spaghetti sauce at the end of cooking plain macaroni and cheese for Pasta Royale – a creamy tomato and cheese sauce.

♦ **Substitute** Mexican flavored cheese and add a large spoon full of salsa at the end for Cheesy Mexican Pasta. Don't forget the jalapenos!

♦ **Substitute** mozzarella style cheese and add a dash of nutmeg for Alfredo Pasta. Add steamed broccoli if desired.

Also try these suggestions with the recipe for Dairy Macaroni and Cheese on the next page.

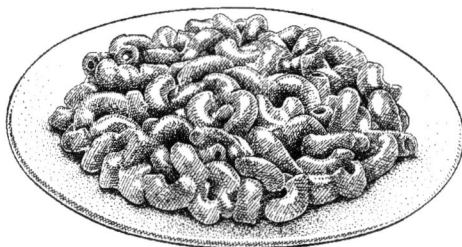

Dairy Mac and Cheese

One pot recipe for dairy cheese and rice pasta

Ingredients:

- 2 oz. brown rice pasta (about 2/3 cup dry pasta)
- 3/4 cup **chicken stock**, *OR* one **chicken bouillon cube** and ¾ cup water
- 3/4 cup milk
- 2 oz. Cheddar, American, or processed cheese
- 1 tsp. **Worcestershire sauce**
- 1/4 tsp. **dry mustard**

Rice Cooker Directions:

Put all ingredients except cheese into the rice cooker. Turn on, cover and stir once in a while. When pasta is almost cooked, about 12 minutes, add the cheese and turn the cooker to warm. Allow the pasta to finish cooking for about 5 minutes. Stir well. Makes 2 portions.

Stovetop Directions:

Put all ingredients except cheese into a 2-quart saucepan on medium heat. Cover and stir once in a while. When pasta is almost cooked, about 12 minutes, add the cheese, cover, and turn off. Allow the pasta to finish cooking for about 5 minutes. Stir well.

Microwave Directions:

In a 2 quart microwavable container, combine pasta, stock and milk. Cook for 8 minutes. Stir, and add cheese and seasonings. Continue cooking for 30 second intervals until cheese is melted. Let rest for 5 minutes. Stir and serve.

Nutrition Information...
Calories: 277   Protein: 13 g   Carbs: 27 g   Fat: 12 g

● ● ● ● ● ● ● ● ● ● ● ● ● ● ● ●

Quick Alfredo Sauce

A rich version of the real thing without the chef

Ingredients:

- ♦ 2 oz. **cream cheese alternative**, or dairy cream cheese
- ♦ 1/3 cup **rice, soy, almond or dairy milk**
- ♦ 1 Tbsp. **soy or dairy Parmesan cheese**
- ♦ 1/4 tsp. garlic powder
- ♦ 1/8 tsp. nutmeg, ground

Rice Cooker or Stovetop Directions:

Combine the cream cheese and milk and warm over low heat, stirring occasionally, until the cream cheese is melted and smooth. Add the Parmesan and spices. Salt to taste. Pour over cooked pasta or use in casseroles. Makes 1 portion.

Microwave Directions:

Combine the cream cheese and milk in a 2 cup microwave safe container. Heat on high for 30 seconds and stir. Stir and heat in 15 second intervals until the cream cheese can be stirred smooth. Add the Parmesan and spices. Pour over cooked pasta. Tip: Can be used in casseroles instead of canned cream soup.

Nutrition Information...
Calories: 266   Protein: 9 g   Carbs: 12 g   Fat: 19 g

*C*reative Cooking:
Add fresh steamed vegetables and cooked pasta spirals for **Pasta Primavera**.
Add bacon and peas with cooked rice noodles for a **Pasta Carbonara**.

Meat Spaghetti Sauce
Two cans and a plan

Ingredients:
- ♦ 1/2 lb. lean ground beef, turkey, or chicken
- ♦ 1 -14 oz. can **Italian style stewed tomato**
- ♦ 1 -8 oz. can **tomato sauce**
- ♦ 1 tsp. basil
- ♦ 1/4 tsp. garlic powder
- ♦ 1/4 tsp. black pepper
- ♦ Salt to taste

Recipe Directions:
On a stovetop or in a rice cooker, brown the ground meat. Drain off any fat and add the rest of the ingredients. Bring to a simmer and cook for 10 - 15 minutes, breaking up the tomatoes. Serve over pasta or noodles. Makes 2 portions.

Nutrition Information:
Calories: 197   Protein: 18 g   Carbs: 15 g   Fat: 8 g

Shopping Tip:
Stewed tomatoes are sweeter than diced tomatoes, and so make a sweeter sauce. If you want to substitute a diced tomato with Italian seasonings, go ahead.

Creative Cooking:
Add in a shake or two of Parmesan cheese, a spoonful of black olive slices, or hot peppers to taste.

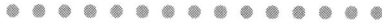

One Pot Pasta in Sauce

*The easiest way to make pasta on the quick – the pasta cooks
right in the sauce*

Ingredients:

- ♦ 2 oz. gluten free rice pasta, dry (about 2/3 cup)
- ♦ 3/4 cup marinara **pasta sauce**
- ♦ 1 cup water

Rice Cooker Directions:

Measure and combine all ingredients in the rice cooker insert.
Turn on. Check pasta, stirring once. When pasta is just reaching
the tender stage (about 15 minutes) cover and turn the rice
cooker to "keep warm" for 5 minutes.

Stovetop Directions:

Measure and combine all ingredients in a 1-quart saucepan on
medium heat. Stir often. When pasta is just tender, turn the heat
off and cover for 5 minutes.

Microwave Directions:

Combine all ingredients in microwave safe bowl. Cover loosely.
Microwave for 8 minutes. Check and stir. Microwave for 2-3
minutes more. Allow to rest for 5 minutes before eating.

Nutrition Information...
Calories: 240   Protein: 5 g   Carbs: 43 g   Fat: 5 g

*S*hopping Tip...
    This recipe works well with rice pastas but not with corn or
    quinoa pasta – they tend to fall apart.
If you use a chunky vegetable pasta sauce, increase the water by
¼ cup.

Baked Ziti

Cheesy tomato sauce with pasta

Ingredients:

- ♦ 2 oz. brown rice pasta (about 2/3 cup dry pasta)
- ♦ 3/4 cup **marinara pasta sauce**
- ♦ 1 cup water
- ♦ 1/4 cup **Italian seasoned tofu**, crumbled; OR, dairy ricotta or cottage cheese
- ♦ 1 oz. shredded **soy cheese** or dairy Mozzarella cheese

Rice Cooker Directions:

Combine water, pasta, and sauce in rice cooker. Turn on and cook for 6-8 minutes. Add the soy cheese. Cook until pasta is almost done. Stir in the tofu or dairy cheeses. Turn rice cooker to off. Let the pasta set for 5 minutes with the cover on. Stir and serve. Makes 2 portions.

Nutrition Analysis:
Calories: 283   Protein: 9 g   Carbs: 46 g   Fat: 7 g

*C*reative Cooking...
    Add Italian seasoning, red pepper flakes, smoked sausage slices, onions or peppers at the beginning of cooking to spice up your ziti.

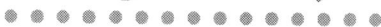

Pizzaria Pasta

Just like a pizza only in a pot...

Ingredients:

- ♦ 2 oz. brown rice pasta (about 2/3 cup dry pasta)
- ♦ 3/4 cup **pizza sauce**
- ♦ 1 cup water
- ♦ 2 oz. **soy cheese**, crumbled, or dairy cheese
- ♦ 1 oz. **pepperoni or smoked sausage**, diced or sliced (OR vegan alternative like soy chorizo)
- ♦ 1 tsp. oregano, dried
- ♦ 1/2 tsp. basil, dried
- ♦ 1 tsp. garlic powder

Rice Cooker Directions:

Combine all ingredients in rice cooker. Turn on to high and cook for 12-15 minutes, stirring once or twice. When pasta is tender, turn to warm and cover for 5 minutes. Makes 2 portions.

Microwave Directions:

Combine all ingredients in a 4 quart microwave safe container. Cook on high for 10-12 minutes, stirring from the bottom once or twice. Keep cooking until pasta is tender and let sit for 2-5 minutes.

Nutrition Information...
Calories 356   Protein: 13 g   Carbs: 48 g   Fat: 13 g

Substitutes...

If using dairy cheese, add it at the last 5 minutes of cooking instead of at the start of cooking.

Creative Cooking...

Add onions, peppers, diced zucchini, olives, or vegetables you like on pizza, *OR*
Add different pasta sauces like chunky vegetable, roasted garlic, or herb.

Bacon Cheeseburger Pasta
Just like a cheeseburger without the bun

Ingredients:
- ½ lb. ground beef (or turkey, chicken)
- 2 slices **cooked bacon**, crumbled
- 1/2 cup **spaghetti sauce**
- 1/4 cup **ketchup**
- 1 tsp. **mustard**
- 2 oz. **shredded soy cheese**
- 1 1/3 cup _cooked_ **brown rice pasta** (penne, elbows, or twists work great) – about 2/3 cup uncooked pasta

Recipe Directions:
Cook pasta and drain.

Brown the ground meat in a medium saucepan, rice cooker or microwave. Drain the fat.

Add the bacon, tomato sauce, ketchup, mustard and cheese. Bring to a simmer and add the cooked pasta stirring gently. Cook for another 2-3 minutes until bubbling and hot. Makes 2 portions.

If using dairy cheese, add it later with the pasta instead of earlier. Soy cheese needs additional time to melt. Makes 2 portions.

Nutrition Information:
Calories: 508   Protein: 31g   Carbs: 42 g   Fat: 22 g

Bacon Ranch Noodles
Tangy flavors make noodles special

Ingredients:
- 2 oz. GF rice noodles
- 1 Tbsp. **bacon bits**
- 1/2 cup **milk or substitute**
- 2 oz. **soy cheese**, shredded or dairy cheese
- 1 Tbsp. dry **Ranch salad dressing mix**

Rice Cooker or Stovetop Directions:
Cook the rice noodles according to the instructions.

In a medium skillet or rice cooker, add the bacon and milk. Bring to a simmer; add the cheese and ranch seasoning. Cook until hot. Add the noodles and cook for 1-2 minutes more. Makes 1 portion.

Nutrition Information:
Calories: 215   Protein: 5 g   Carbs: 31 g   Fat: 7 g

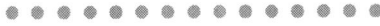

Beef Broccoli Noodles

Easier than take-out

Ingredients:

- 2 oz. GF rice noodles
- 8 oz. beef stir fry meat, cut in thin strips (or **seasoned tofu**)
- 2 Tbsp. vegetable oil
- 1/4 cup orange juice
- 1 tsp. **beef or vegetable bouillon**
- 2 cups broccoli, raw, chopped
- 1 Tbsp. **soy sauce or tamari**
- ¼ tsp. crushed red pepper

Rice Cooker or Stovetop Directions:

Cook the rice noodles according to the instructions.

In a medium skillet or rice cooker, heat the oil and brown the beef strips. To the skillet, add the broccoli, orange juice, and bouillon. Bring to a simmer and add the noodles. When broccoli is bright green, add the soy sauce or tamari and pepper. Stir until well combined. Makes 2 portions.

Nutrition Information:
Calories: 454   Protein: 30 g   Carbs: 31 g   Fat: 24 g

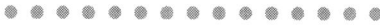

Beef Chili Noodles

Love chili? You will love these noodles

Ingredients:

- ♦ 2 oz. GF rice noodles
- ♦ 1/2 lb. ground beef (or ground turkey, chicken, **seasoned tofu**)
- ♦ 1 -8 oz. can **tomato sauce**
- ♦ 1 Tbsp. **chili seasoning mix**
- ♦ 1 cup **kidney beans**, drained

Rice Cooker or Stovetop Directions:

Cook the rice noodles according to the instructions.
In a medium skillet or rice cooker, crumble the ground meat and cook on medium heat until the meat is browned. Pour off the fat. To the skillet, add the chili seasoning mix, tomato sauce and kidney beans. When hot, add the noodles. Stir until well combined. Makes 2 portions.

Nutrition Information:
Calories: 457   Protein: 33 g   Carbs: 53 g   Fat: 12 g

*S*hopping Tip...
What to do with a half can of leftover kidney beans? Marinate with Italian dressing and other vegetables for a great salad the next day. Or, cook with rice and a couple of spoonfuls of salsa and chili seasoning for a quick red beans and rice.

Cheesy Corn Noodles

Creamy noodles with a crunch for the corn lover

Ingredients:
- ♦ 2 oz. GF rice noodles
- ♦ 1 -8 oz. can **creamed corn**
- ♦ 2 oz. meltable **soy or dairy cheese**
- ♦ ¼ cup corn chips, crushed

Rice Cooker or Stovetop Directions:
Cook the rice noodles according to the instructions.
In a medium skillet or rice cooker, heat the creamed corn. When hot, add the cheese and stir until melted. Add the noodles and continue cooking until hot. Serve with the crumbled corn chips on top. Makes 1 portion.

Microwave Directions:
Cook the rice noodles according to the instructions.
In a 2 quart microwave container, combine the creamed corn and cheese. Microwave for 3-4 minutes and stir. Continue to microwave in 30 second intervals until the cheese has melted. Add the noodles and cook for 1-2 more minutes. Serve with the crumbled corn chips on top. Makes 1 portion.

Nutrition Information:
Calories: 299   Protcin: 6 g   Carbs: 53 g   Fat: 8 g

Beef Mushroom Noodles
Beef stroganoff in one dish

Ingredients:
- 2 oz. GF rice noodles
- 1/2 lb. ground beef (or turkey, chicken, seasoned tofu)
- 2 Tbsp. water
- 1 Tbsp. dried minced onion
- 1 tsp. **beef bouillon**
- 1 tsp. garlic powder
- 1 can mushrooms, drained
- 1 whole tomato, diced
- 2 Tbsp. non-dairy or dairy **sour cream**

Rice Cooker or Stovetop Directions:
Cook the rice noodles according to the instructions.

In a medium skillet or rice cooker, crumble the ground beef and cook on medium heat until the meat is browned. Pour off the fat. To the skillet, add the bouillon, onion flakes, garlic powder, water and noodles. When hot, add the sour cream and tomato. Stir until well combined. Makes 2 portions.

Nutrition Information:
Calories: 383   Protein: 27 g   Carbs: 36 g   Fat: 15 g

Brat Coins and Peppers with Noodles
Sausage and peppers with filling pasta –
a hungry student's fuel

Ingredients:
♦ 2 oz. GF rice noodles
♦ 1 tsp. vegetable oil
♦ 1 small green pepper, sliced
♦ 1 link **bratwurst**, heat & serve (or **cooked sausage** link)
♦ 1 Tbsp. **honey mustard**

Rice Cooker or Stovetop Directions:
Cook the rice noodles according to the instructions.
In a medium skillet or rice cooker, add the oil and peppers. While the peppers are cooking, cut the cooked bratwurst into ¼" coins. Add to the skillet. Continue cooking until peppers are tender. Add the noodles and cook until hot. Drizzle honey mustard over noodles, toss quickly, and eat. Makes 1 portion.

Microwave Instructions:
Cook the rice noodles according to the instructions.
In a 2 quart microwave container, combine sausage coins, oil and peppers. Cook on high for 4-5 minutes or until peppers are just soft. Add the noodles and honey mustard and toss. Cook for 1-2 minutes more. Makes 1 portion.

Nutrition Information:
Calories: 272   Protein: 8 g   Carbs: 29 g   Fat: 14 g

● ● ● ● ● ● ● ● ● ● ● ● ● ● ●

Cheddar Beef Noodle Skillet

Cheesy beef and tomato one dish meal

Ingredients:

- ♦ 2 oz. GF rice noodles
- ♦ 1/2 lb. ground beef (or turkey, chicken, seasoned tofu)
- ♦ 1 -8 oz. can corn, drained
- ♦ 8 oz. **tomato sauce**
- ♦ 1 tsp. **beef or vegetable bouillon**
- ♦ 2 oz. Cheddar style **soy or dairy cheese**

Rice Cooker or Stovetop Directions:

Cook the rice noodles according to the instructions.

In a medium skillet or rice cooker, crumble the ground beef and cook on medium heat until the meat is browned. Pour off the fat into a container. Add the bouillon, drained corn, tomato sauce, the cheese and noodles. Heat until bubbly. Makes 2 portions.

Nutrition Information:
Calories: 494   Protein: 34 g   Carbs: 41 g   Fat: 21 g

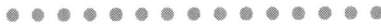

Cheeseburger Rice Noodles

*Quick cheeseburger taste that's just as filling
as with the bun*

Ingredients:

- ♦ 2 oz. GF rice noodles
- ♦ 1/2 lb. ground beef (or turkey, chicken, seasoned tofu)
- ♦ 1 tsp. **beef bouillon**
- ♦ 2 Tbsp. water
- ♦ 2 oz. meltable **soy cheese** or dairy American cheese
- ♦ 1 whole tomato, diced

Rice Cooker or Stovetop Directions:

Cook the rice noodles according to the instructions.

In a medium skillet or rice cooker, crumble the ground beef and cook on medium heat until the meat is browned. Pour off the fat into a container. Add the bouillon, water and noodles. When hot, add the cheese and tomato. Stir until the cheese is melted. Makes 2 portions.

If desired, finish with 2 tablespoons salsa for a Mexican flavor.

Nutrition Information:
Calories: 428   Protein: 32 g   Carbs: 26 g   Fat: 21 g

Chicken Cacciatore Noodles

Cheesy chicken and tomato meal...

Ingredients:

- ◆ 2 oz. GF rice noodles
- ◆ 3/4 cup chunky **spaghetti sauce**
- ◆ 1 cup water
- ◆ 1- 5 oz. can **chicken**, canned with broth
- ◆ 1/4 small green pepper, diced or strips
- ◆ 1/2 small onion, diced or strips
- ◆ 1/2 tsp. **Italian seasoning**
- ◆ 2 oz. **soy cheese** or dairy cheese

Rice Cooker or Stovetop Directions:

Cook the rice noodles according to the instructions.
Combine the rest of the ingredients except cheese. Cover and turn on (medium heat). Simmer for 15 minutes or until the peppers are tender. Add the cheese and melt. Serve over the noodles, or toss together. Top with Parmesan if desired. Makes 2 portions.

Nutrition Information...
Calories: 410   Protein: 25 g   Carbs: 50 g   Fat: 13 g

Creative Cooking...

Add crushed red pepper flakes for spice, *OR*
Add one spoonful of sour cream or cream cheese at the end for creamier tasting pasta.

Shopping Tip...

Choose a chunky vegetable spaghetti sauce over plain marinara – the flavor and extras are already in it.

Substitutions...

You can substitute cooked chicken cut in strips (3-4 oz.) or sliced seasoned tofu for the canned chicken in this recipe.

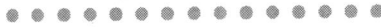

Chicken Alfredo Noodles

Add vegetables like broccoli, shredded carrot, and diced tomato for Pasta Primavera.

Ingredients:

- 2 oz. GF rice noodles
- 1/2 cup **rice, soy, almond or dairy milk**
- 1 oz. **non-dairy or dairy cream cheese**
- 5 oz. **canned chicken**, drained, or 1/3 cup cooked chicken, diced
- 1/2 tsp. **chicken or vegetable bouillon**
- 1 tsp. parsley flakes
- 1/4 tsp. **Italian seasoning**
- 2 Tbsp. **Parmesan soy cheese**, or substitute

Rice Cooker or Stovetop Directions:

Cook the rice noodles according to the instructions.
In a medium skillet or rice cooker, add the milk, cream cheese and bouillon, stirring well. When the cream cheese has melted, add the chicken meat, vegetables if using, and seasonings. Bring to a simmer and add the noodles. Top with the Parmesan and serve. Makes 2 portions.

Microwave Directions:

Cook the rice noodles according to the instructions.
In a 2 quart microwave container, add the milk, cream cheese, and bouillon. Cook for 1 minute and stir. When the cream cheese has melted, add the bouillon, chicken meat, vegetables if using, and seasonings. Cook for 4-6 minutes and add the noodles. Stir. Heat for another minute. Top with the Parmesan and serve. Makes 2 portions.

Nutrition Information:
Calories: 277   Protein: 19 g   Carbs: 32 g   Fat: 8 g

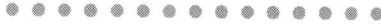

Chicken Fajita Noodles
The flavor of fajitas with quick noodles

Ingredients:
- 2 oz. GF rice noodles
- 1 tsp. vegetable oil
- 1 cup **fajita vegetable blend**, fresh or frozen
- 1 -5 oz. can **chicken**, drained; or **seasoned tofu**
- 2 tsp. **taco seasoning mix**

Rice Cooker or Stovetop Directions:
Cook the rice noodles according to the instructions.
In a medium skillet or rice cooker, add the oil and sauté the fajita vegetables until hot. Add the chicken meat and taco seasoning. Cook until the chicken is hot. Mix in the noodles. Makes 2 portions.

Microwave Directions.
Cook the rice noodles according to the instructions.
In a 2 quart microwave container, toss the vegetables with the oil. Microwave for 3 minutes, or until the vegetables start to soften. Add the chicken meat and taco seasoning. Stir and cook until the chicken is hot. Mix in the noodles. Cook for 1-2 minutes more. Makes 2 portions.

Top off with sour cream or salsa.

Nutrition Information:
Calories: 196   Protein: 14 g   Carbs: 30 g   Fat: 3 g

Chicken Curry Noodles

*You can use any kind of gluten free curry power in this recipe.
Curry powders are usually seven or more spices combined to be
called curry. They come in all kinds of "heat" as well. The Asian red
paste is spicier than the green. Start with 1/4 teaspoon and work
your way up!*

Ingredients:

- ♦ 2 oz. GF rice noodles
- ♦ 1 tsp. **chicken or vegetable bouillon**
- ♦ 1 cup **rice, soy, almond or dairy milk**
- ♦ 1 Tbsp. cornstarch
- ♦ 1 tsp. **green curry paste**
- ♦ 1 -5 oz. can **chicken**, drained; or **seasoned tofu**
- ♦ 1/2 cup green peas, frozen (optional)

Recipe Directions:

Cook the rice noodles according to the instructions.

In a medium skillet or rice cooker, add the cornstarch and stir in
the rice milk until the cornstarch is dissolved. Then stir in the
bouillon and curry paste. Bring to a simmer and add the chicken
meat and peas. Continue cooking until thick and hot. Stir in the
noodles. Makes 2 portions.

Nutrition Information:
Calories: 255   Protein: 15 g   Carbs: 39 g   Fat: 5 g

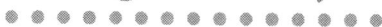

Noodles with Gravy

Add frozen peas, drained canned mushrooms or other vegetables as the gravy cooks.

Ingredients:
- ♦ 2 oz. GF rice noodles
- ♦ 2 tsp. cornstarch or potato starch
- ♦ 1 tsp. **beef or vegetable bouillon**
- ♦ 1 tsp. **margarine** or butter
- ♦ 3/4 cup water

Recipe Directions:
Cook the rice noodles according to the instructions.

Rice Cooker or Stovetop Directions:
In a saucepan, add the corn or potato starch. Stir in the water. Add the bouillon and margarine.
Bring to a boil (add vegetables now if desired) and cook for 3-5 minutes until thick and clear. Add the noodles and heat one minute longer. Makes 1 portion.

Microwave Directions:
In a 2 quart microwave container, add the corn or potato starch. Stir in the water. Add the bouillon and margarine.
Cook for 1 minute on high, stir and cook in 30 second intervals until thick and clear. Add noodles and cook for 30 seconds more. Makes 1 portion.

Nutrition Information:
Calories: 258   Protein: 3 g   Carbs: 52 g   Fat: 4 g

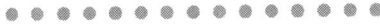

Chicken Lo Mein Noodles

Spice it up with a teaspoon of Asian chili sauce, garlic blend seasoning, or a squeeze of lemon and a drizzle of honey.

Ingredients:

- 2 oz. GF rice noodles
- 1 tsp. **chicken or vegetable bouillon**
- 1/2 cup water
- 1/2 cup green pepper, chopped
- 6 baby carrots, sliced
- 1 small onion, diced
- 5 oz. canned **chicken**, drained; or 1/2 cup **seasoned tofu**
- 1 Tbsp. **soy sauce or tamari**

Recipe Directions:

Cook the rice noodles according to the instructions.

In a medium skillet or rice cooker, add the water, onion, pepper, carrot and bouillon. Bring to a simmer and cook until the carrot is almost tender. Add the chicken meat, the noodles and the soy sauce or tamari. Continue cooking until hot. Makes 2 portions.

Nutrition Information:
Calories: 214   Protein: 16 g   Carbs: 32 g   Fat: 3 g

Chinese Fried Noodles

Take out at home

Ingredients:

- 2 oz. GF rice noodles
- 1 tsp. canola oil, cold pressed
- 3/4 cups **oriental vegetables**, fresh or frozen
- 1/2 tsp. **beef or vegetable bouillon**
- 1 Tbsp. **soy sauce or tamari**
- 1 large egg
- ½ tsp. sesame seeds (optional)
- 1 green onion, sliced (optional)

Recipe Directions:

Cook the rice noodles according to the instructions.

In a medium skillet, heat the oil. Add the vegetables and cook until almost tender. Add the bouillon, soy sauce or tamari, and noodles. When hot, beat the egg and drizzle over the noodles. Quickly move the noodles around so the egg cooks. Continue cooking until all the egg is solid. Sprinkle with sesame seeds or sliced green onions if desired. Makes 1 portion.

Nutrition Information:
Calories: 356   Protein: 12 g   Carbs: 52 g   Fat: 10 g

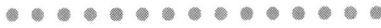

Creamy Chicken and Broccoli Noodles

Comfort food at its best

Ingredients:

- ♦ 2 oz. GF rice noodles
- ♦ 1 -5 oz. can **chicken**, drained; or **cannellini beans**
- ♦ 1/3 cup water
- ♦ 2 cups broccoli, raw, chopped
- ♦ 1 tsp. **chicken or vegetable bouillon**
- ♦ 2 Tbsp. **sour cream alternative** or dairy sour cream

Recipe Directions:

Cook the rice noodles according to the instructions.

Rice Cooker or Stovetop Directions:
In a medium skillet or rice cooker, add the cooked chicken (or vegan substitute), water, broccoli, and bouillon. Bring to a simmer and cook until the broccoli is bright green. Add the noodles and sour cream. Stir until well combined. Makes 2 portions.

Microwave Directions:
In a 2 quart microwave safe container, combine the chicken, water, broccoli, and bouillon. Cook for 3 minutes, covered and vented. Stir in the sour cream. Add the noodles and cook for 2 more minutes or until hot. Let rest for 3-4 minutes and stir. Makes 2 portions.

Nutrition Information:
Calories: 251   Protein: 17 g   Carbs: 35 g   Fat: 6 g

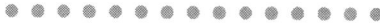

Green Bean Casserole Noodles

Just like the holiday casserole, only anytime of the year

Ingredients:

- ♦ 2 oz. GF rice noodles
- ♦ 1/2 cup **rice, soy, almond or dairy milk**
- ♦ 2 Tbsp. **cream cheese alternative** or dairy cream cheese
- ♦ 1 oz. meltable **soy cheese** or dairy cheese
- ♦ 1 Tbsp. **onion soup mix**
- ♦ 1/2 cup green beans, frozen
- ♦ 1/4 cup **potato chips**, crushed (one small bag)

Recipe Directions:

Cook the rice noodles according to the instructions.

In a medium skillet or rice cooker, heat the rice milk, cream cheese, American cheese and onion soup mix. Stir to melt the cheeses. Add the green beans and noodles. Cook until hot. Serve with the crumbled potato chips on top. Makes 1 portion.

Nutrition Information:
Calories: 235   Protein: 4 g   Carbs: 37 g   Fat: 7 g

● ● ● ● ● ● ● ● ● ● ● ● ● ●

Spicy Peanut Noodles

A quick version of the classic take out meal...

Ingredients:

- 2 oz. GF rice noodles
- 2 Tbsp. smooth **peanut butter** or sunflower butter
- 1/2 tsp. toasted sesame oil
- 1 Tbsp. **soy sauce or tamari**
- 1/2 packet sugar, or other sweetener
- 1/4 tsp. **Thai sweet chili sauce** (optional)
- 1 stalk green onion (optional)

Rice Cooker Directions:

Heat 3 cups of water to boiling in the rice cooker and put in 1/4 the package of rice sticks. Turn to warm. Soak for 10 minutes. While the noodles are soaking, mix together the peanut butter, sesame oil, soy sauce or tamari, and hot sauce. Drain the noodles and put back into the rice cooker insert with 2 tablespoons of water. Turn on high and heat until noodles are warm. Add the sauce and green onion and stir. Cook until sauce sticks to noodles. Makes 1 large portion.

Microwave Directions:

Heat 3 cups of water to boiling in a 4 quart microwavable container, and put in 1/4 the package of rice sticks, cook for 4 minutes. Soak for 5 minutes more. While the noodles are soaking, mix together the peanut butter, sesame oil, soy sauce or tamari, and hot sauce. Drain the noodles, and mix with the sauce and 1 tablespoons of water. Heat until noodles are hot, about 2-4 minutes. Add the green onion and stir. Eat right away. Makes 1 large portion.

Nutrition Information...
Calories 445   Protein: 12 g   Carbs: 56 g   Fat: 21 g

*C*reative Cooking...
Add cooked oriental vegetables or bean sprouts, diced cooked chicken, turkey, tofu, beef, pork, or sausage. Thai chili sauce, fresh squeezed lime juice, or lemon grass seasoning add authentic flavor.

Cheesy Tuna Noodles

The gluten free version of tuna noodle casserole...

Ingredients:

- ◆ 3/4 cup **chicken or vegetable stock**
- ◆ 2 oz. GF rice noodles, broken into 2" pieces
- ◆ 1 small can mushrooms, drained
- ◆ 2 oz. meltable **soy cheese** or dairy cheese
- ◆ 1- 5oz. can **tuna**, drained

Rice Cooker Directions:

Heat the stock in the rice cooker. Add broken up noodles (rice sticks) and the drained mushrooms. When the stock begins to bubble, add the soy cheese and cook for another 4-5 minutes, stirring occasionally. If you want to use dairy cheese instead of soy cheese, add it the last one minute of cooking. Stir in the drained tuna and cook for another 2 minutes. Season with salt and pepper to taste. Makes 2 portions.

Microwave Directions:

In a 2 quart microwavable container, cook the stock on high for 2 minutes. Add the mushrooms, rice noodles (broken into 1" pieces), and soy cheese. Cook on high covered loosely for 6-8 minutes until the pasta is tender and the soy cheese is melted. If you want to use dairy cheese instead of soy cheese, add it the last one minute of cooking. Stir in the drained tuna and stir. Cook for 1 minute more. Allow to cool for 2 minutes. Stir, season and serve. Makes 2 portions.

Nutrition Information...
Calories 307   Protein: 27 g   Carbs: 27g   Fat: 8 g

*C*reative Cooking...
　　Add your choice of vegetables at the beginning of cooking
　　- peas, onions, red peppers or pimentos.
Add a seasoning blend, dash of dill weed, or splash of hot sauce.

Ham and Cheese Noodles

Add a vegetable like peas, green beans, or corn at the start of cooking. Add a drizzle of honey mustard at the end for additional flavor.

Ingredients:

- ◆ 2 oz. GF rice noodles
- ◆ 4 oz. **ham**, diced
- ◆ 1/2 cup **rice, soy, almond or dairy milk**
- ◆ 2 oz. meltable **soy cheese,** or dairy cheese

Recipe Directions:

Cook the rice noodles according to the instructions.

In a medium skillet or rice cooker, add the ham and milk. Bring to a simmer, add the cheese, and cook until hot. Add the noodles. Makes 1 portion.

Nutrition Information:
Calories: 279   Protein: 14 g   Carbs: 30 g   Fat: 10 g

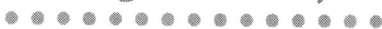

Pizza Noodle Casserole

Craving pizza? This dish will satisfy

Ingredients:

- ♦ 4 oz. GF rice noodles
- ♦ 1 small can mushrooms, drained
- ♦ 15 slices **pepperoni**; or vegan alternative
- ♦ 1 cup **pizza sauce** (or 2/3 of a 14 oz. can)
- ♦ 2 oz. mozzarella style **soy cheese**, or dairy Mozzarella

Recipe Directions:

Preheat an oven or toaster oven to 350° degrees F. Cook rice noodles as directed on package and drain well. Combine noodles, mushrooms, pepperoni, and the pizza sauce in a bowl and turn into a greased ovenproof baking dish (8"x8" inch square or 8" round pan works well). Top with the cheese. Bake for 25-30 minutes or until the cheese is melted. Makes 2 portions.

Nutrition Information:
Calories: 463   Protein: 12 g   Carbs: 60 g   Fat: 18 g

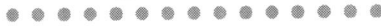

Sausage and Spice Noodles

Real Italian flavor with the heat of the southwest

Ingredients:

- ♦ 2 oz. GF rice noodles
- ♦ 4 oz. **Italian ground sausage,** or soy **Chorizo**
- ♦ 1/2 small onion, diced
- ♦ 1/2 small green pepper, diced
- ♦ 3/4 cup salsa (hot as you want)

Recipe Directions:

Cook the rice noodles according to the instructions.

In a medium skillet or rice cooker, crumble the Italian sausage and add the onions and peppers. Cook on medium heat until the meat is browned. Pour off the fat into a container to dispose of latter when cool. To the skillet add the salsa and noodles. Stir until well combined. Makes 1 portion.

Nutrition Information:
Calories: 306   Protein: 10 g   Carbs: 37 g   Fat: 13 g

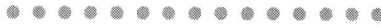

Tomato Soup Noodles

As comfortable as Cream of Tomato Soup

Ingredients:

♦ 4 oz. GF rice noodles
♦ 1/2 cup **rice, soy, almond or dairy milk**
♦ 1 tsp. **beef, chicken, or vegetable bouillon**
♦ 2/3 cup **spaghetti sauce**
♦ 1/2 tsp. sugar (optional)
♦ 1/8 cup **soy Parmesan cheese** or dairy Parmesan

Recipe Directions:

Cook the rice noodles according to the instructions.

Rice Cooker or Stovetop Directions:

In a medium saucepan over medium heat, mix the milk, bouillon, pasta sauce, and sugar together. Stir occasionally. When hot, add the noodles. Simmer for about 5 minutes. Let rest for 2-3 minutes. Stir and serve with Parmesan cheese. Makes 2 portions.

Microwave Directions:

In a 2 quart microwave container, mix the milk, bouillon, pasta sauce, and sugar together. Cook covered and vented for 3-4 minutes. Stir occasionally. When hot, add the noodles. Cook 2-3 minutes more or until hot. Let rest for 2-3 minutes. Stir and serve with Parmesan cheese. Makes 2 portions.

Nutrition Information:
Calories: 412   Protein: 18 g   Carbs: 62 g   Fat: 9 g

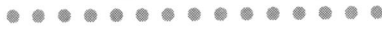

Tuna Noodle Casserole

A standard for all students

Ingredients:
- 2 oz. GF rice noodles
- 1/2 cup **rice, soy, almond or dairy milk**
- 1 oz. **non-dairy or dairy cream cheese**
- 2 slices **soy cheese**, or dairy cheese
- 1 -4 oz. can **tuna** in water, drained
- 1 tsp. parsley flakes
- 1/2 oz. **potato chips**, crushed (one small bag)

Recipe Directions:
Cook the rice noodles according to the instructions.

In a medium skillet or rice cooker, add the rice milk and cream cheese. Stir and when the cream cheese has melted, add the cheese slices, tuna, and parsley. Bring to a simmer and add the noodles. Pour into a small casserole dish and top with the crushed potato chips.

Bake at 350° degrees F. for 15 - 20 minutes in a regular or toaster oven. To microwave instead of bake, cover the casserole with wax paper and cook for 6 minutes on 70% power. Makes 1 portion.

Nutrition Information:
Calories: 356   Protein: 21 g   Carbs: 34 g   Fat: 13 g

Tuscan Chicken Noodles

A light pasta dish ready in a minute

Ingredients:

♦   2 oz. GF rice noodles
♦   ½- 14 oz. can **diced tomato** w/basil, garlic & oregano
♦   1- 5 oz. can canned **chicken**, drained; or **seasoned tofu**
♦   1/4 tsp. **Italian seasoning**

Recipe Directions:

Cook the rice noodles according to the instructions.

Rice Cooker or Stovetop Directions:

In a medium skillet or rice cooker, add the tomatoes, chicken meat, and seasoning. Bring to a simmer and cook until hot. Add the noodles. Serve with Parmesan if desired. Makes 1 portion.

Microwave Directions:

In a 2-quart microwave safe container, mix together the tomatoes, chicken meat and seasoning. Cook covered and vented for 4 minutes. Add the noodles and continue cooking for 2-3 minutes. Stir and let rest for 5 minutes. Top with Parmesan cheese if desired.

Nutrition Information:
Calories: 380   Protein: 15 g   Carbs: 58 g   Fat: 6 g

Beef and a Side Noodles
A hearty Midwestern style meal

Ingredients:
- ♦ 2 oz. GF rice noodles or pasta
- ♦ 1/2 lb. ground beef (or turkey, turkey sausage, chicken)
- ♦ 1 -8 oz. can **tomato sauce**
- ♦ 1 cup mixed vegetables, frozen
- ♦ 1 tsp. **beef bouillon**

Recipe Directions:
Cook the rice noodles according to the instructions.

In a medium skillet or rice cooker, crumble the ground beef and cook on medium heat until the meat is browned. Pour off the fat into a container. To the skillet or cooker, add the bouillon, tomato sauce and vegetables. When hot, add the cooked noodles. Stir until well combined and hot. Makes 2 portions.

Nutrition Information:
Calories: 384 Protein: 28 g   Carbs: 40 g   Fat: 12 g

*C*reative Cooking...
Spice it up with taco seasoning, chili powder, or garlic blend seasoning - start with 1/4 teaspoon and add to taste.

Rice

Faster than takeout and half the price

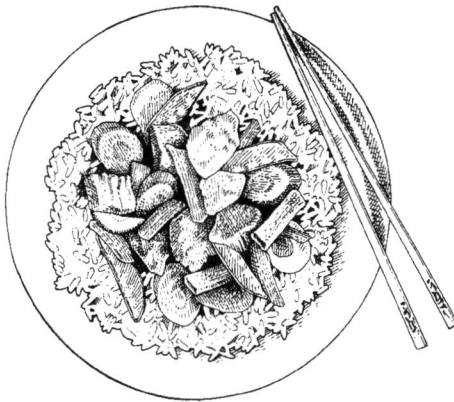

Rice for One

Cooking rice as a side or for a casserole is
quick and easy in the microwave

Ingredients:
- ♦ 1 cup water
- ♦ 1/4 cup white rice

Microwave Instructions:

In a 1-quart glass measuring cup or bowl, stir together 1 cup water with white rice (use 1-1/4 cups with brown rice). Cook, uncovered, in a microwave oven at full power until most of the water is absorbed, 10 to 11 minutes (20 minutes for brown rice).

Cover with plastic wrap and continue cooking at half power (50 percent) until tender, 2 to 5 minutes longer. Add salt to taste.

Nutrition Information...
Calories: 168   Protein: 3 g   Carbs: 37 g   Fat: 1 g

Instant Chicken Rice Soup
Comfort food that's between classes fast

Ingredients:
- 1 tsp. **chicken bouillon** (or one cube)
- 2 Tbsp. **instant brown or white rice**
- 1/2 tsp. parsley flakes
- 1/4 tsp. onion powder
- 1 cup water

Recipe Directions:

Combine all ingredients and microwave for 4 minutes. Stir and cover for 3-4 minutes. Stir again and enjoy.

Nutrition Information:
Calories: 108   Protein: 3 g   Carbs: 22 g   Fat: 1 g

Note: Items listed in **bold** in the recipes have a higher incidence of containing gluten – it's a *reminder* to always check the label or directly with the manufacturer.

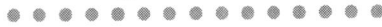

Fast Spanish Rice

A single serving of seasoned rice – a great snack

Ingredients:

- ♦ 1/4 cup instant white or brown rice
- ♦ 1 -6 oz. can **tomato juice**
- ♦ 1/4 cup water
- ♦ 1 tsp. **taco seasoning mix**

Rice Cooker Instructions:

Combine all ingredients in rice cooker and turn on. Cook until the rice absorbs most of the tomato. Let rest on warm for 3-5 minutes. Makes 1 portion.

Stovetop Instructions:

Combine all ingredients in a small saucepan and turn on medium heat. Cook until the rice absorbs most of the tomato. Turn off and cover for 3-5 minutes. Makes 1 portion.

Microwave Instructions:

Combine all ingredients in covered and vented microwave safe bowl. Cook on high for 6 minutes or until the rice absorbs most of the tomato. Let rest for 3-5 minutes. Makes 1 portion.

Nutrition Information:
Calories: 211   Protein: 5 g   Carbs: 44 g   Fat: 2 g

• • • • • • • • • • • • • • • • •

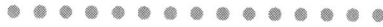

Speed Risotto
A quick microwave version of the classic dish

Ingredients:
- 1/2 cup Arborio or sushi rice
- 1 Tbsp. olive oil
- 1 Tbsp. dried minced onion
- 1 ½ cup **chicken stock**
- 1/4 cup non-dairy or dairy **Parmesan cheese**

Recipe Directions:
In a 2-quart microwave safe container covered, microwave the oil, onion and rice for 4 minutes. Add the chicken broth and cook on high for 16 minutes (covered and vented). Stir and cook for 2 more minutes or until the liquid is almost absorbed. Remove from the microwave and stir. Add the cheese and season as you like with salt, pepper, herb blends. For a creamier risotto, stir in a little milk. Makes 2 portions.

Nutrition Information:
Calories: 294   Protein: 10 g   Carbs: 39 g   Fat: 11 g

C reative Cooking...
Great for a late night snack with raisins and cinnamon stirred in.
Season it up... Add herb mixtures like Italian seasoning, garlic blends, or hot sauce.

Tex-Mex Rice

*Serve with shredded cheese on top, or with corn chip dippers.
Leftover rice makes a great wrap the next day for lunch.*

Ingredients:
- 1 cup white rice
- 1 tsp. **chicken or vegetable bouillon**
- 1 cup water
- 1 -14 oz. can **diced tomato** w/green chilies
- 1 -8 oz. can corn, drained
- 1 small can black olives, sliced
- 1/4 tsp. hot pepper sauce

Recipe Directions:
In a medium saucepan or rice cooker, cook the white rice with the water and bouillon, covered, on medium heat until the water is almost absorbed. Add the diced tomatoes and juice, drained corn, and drained olives. Season with salt and pepper if desired. Stir well, and continue cooking until rice is bubbly hot. Makes 2 portions.

Nutrition Information:
Calories: 264   Protein: 5 g   Carbs: 53 g   Fat: 3 g

Cheesed-Up Spanish Rice

Rich and gooey, this recipe will fill you up

Ingredients:

- 1 cup white rice
- 1 cup water
- 6 oz. shredded white **soy cheese**, or dairy jack cheese
- 1 -12 oz. jar salsa
- 1 -8 oz. can corn, drained
- 1/2 cup **non-dairy or dairy sour cream**

Recipe Directions:

Cook rice in the water using a rice cooker or saucepan. Cool to room temperature.

Combine the cooked rice, half the shredded cheese, half the salsa, drained corn, and the sour cream. Pour into a greased 8"x 8" microwavable or ovenproof dish. Top with the remaining salsa, spreading it evenly over the surface. Sprinkle the remaining cheese over the top. Microwave, covered and vented, for 12-16 minutes. *OR,* Bake in a preheated 350° degree toaster oven or regular oven for 20-25 minutes. Makes 4 portions, or 2 mega portions.

Nutrition Information:
Calories: 351   Protein: 13 g   Carbs: 30 g   Fat: 20 g

Pineapple Ham with Rice
Tangy sweet and sour flavors brighten up ham

Ingredients:
- ♦ 1 tsp. canola oil
- ♦ 1 -5 oz. can **diced ham,** drained; or 1/3 cup **turkey ham,** diced
- ♦ 1 -4 oz. container pineapple tidbits in juice (snack size)
- ♦ 2 Tbsp. **soy sauce or tamari**
- ♦ 1 Tbsp. honey
- ♦ 1 1/2 Tbsp. cornstarch or potato starch
- ♦ 1 cup white rice, *cooked*

Recipe Directions:
Cook rice according to the package directions. Keep warm.

Drain the juice from the canned pineapple and reserve. In a small saucepan or rice cooker, heat the oil and cook the ham until it starts to brown. Add the juice from the pineapple, soy sauce or tamari, and honey. Bring to a boil. Add the pineapple. In a separate bowl, mix the cornstarch with 2 tablespoons water until dissolved. Pour into the ham mixture, stirring often, and cook until thick -- about 3-4 minutes. Serve over the cooked rice. Makes 1 large portion, or two small.

Nutrition Information:
Calories: 680   Protein: 35 g   Carbs: 118 g   Fat: 9 g

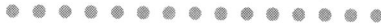

Red Beans and Rice

A Southern favorite made easy

Ingredients:
- 1/4 small onion, raw
- 2 strips celery, sliced
- 1 tsp. vegetable oil
- 1/2 cup white rice, uncooked
- 1/2 tsp. garlic powder
- 1 cup **chicken or vegetable stock**
- 1/2 cup canned **kidney beans**, drained (about 1/2 can)
- 2 Tbsp. salsa
- 1/4 tsp. **hot pepper sauce**

Rice Cooker or Stovetop Directions:
In a medium saucepan or rice cooker, heat the oil and cook the diced onion and sliced celery. Stir and cook until the vegetables start to appear soft. Add the rest of the ingredients and cook until the rice is done. Makes 2 portions.

Microwave Directions:
Combine all ingredients in a one quart covered microwave container and vent. Cook on high for 8 minutes. Stir and cook for 4-6 minutes more, or until rice is cooked.

Nutrition Information:
Calories: 273   Protein: 10 g   Carbs: 46 g   Fat: 5 g

Sloppy Jose Rice

*No need for a bun,
Mexican flavor Sloppy Joe's and rice*

Ingredients:
- 1/2 lb ground beef (or turkey, chicken, seasoned tofu)
- 1 Tbsp. dried minced onion
- 1 -8 oz. can **tomato juice**
- 1/2 cup water
- 1/2 cup white rice
- 1 small green pepper, diced
- 1 cube **beef or vegetable bouillon** (1 tsp. granulated)
- 1/2 tsp. chili powder
- 1/4 cup salsa
- 1/4 cup **ketchup**

Recipe Directions:
In a medium skillet or rice cooker, brown the ground beef and pour off the fat. Add the onion flakes, tomato juice, water, rice, bouillon, chili pepper, and peppers to the pan. Cover and simmer until most of the liquid is absorbed. Add the salsa and ketchup to the pan. Bring back to bubbling and serve. Makes 2 portions.

Nutrition Information:
Calories: 310   Protein: 19 g   Carbs: 39 g   Fat: 8 g

C reative Cooking...
Add corn or other fresh vegetables with the tomato juice, or
Top with sour cream, or guacamole, or
Serve over a bed of corn chips for dipping like nachos, or
Stuff green pepper halves for stuffed peppers - microwave for 4 minutes covered and vented.

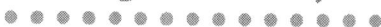

Pizza Rice

Make rice an event...

Ingredients:
- ♦ 1/2 cup white rice, long grain
- ♦ 1/3 cup **pizza sauce**
- ♦ 1 cup water
- ♦ 8 slices **pepperoni**, diced; or **seasoned tofu**
- ♦ 1 oz. **soy cheese**, mozzarella style or dairy mozzarella

Rice Cooker Directions:
Combine rice, pizza sauce, water, and pepperoni in rice cooker. Stir once in a while. Cook until rice cooker turns to low. Sprinkle cheese on top, cover, and enjoy in 5 minutes when the cheese has melted. Makes 2 portions.

Microwave Directions:
Combine rice, pizza sauce, and water in a one quart microwave container. Cook on high for 10 minutes. Add pepperoni and cheese - stir. Continue cooking on high for 3-6 minutes or until rice tests done.

Nutrition Information...
Calories: 280   Protein: 8 g   Carbs: 45 g   Fat: 6 g

*C*reative Cooking...
Add fresh diced onions, peppers, zucchini, or sliced olives.
Stuff pepper halves with rice mixture, drizzle with tomato sauce, and microwave for 4 minutes for quick stuffed peppers.
Spread a wrap with refried beans and fill with pizza rice.
Instead of white rice, use brown rice and 1 cup more water.

*S*hopping Tip...
Choosing turkey pepperoni over regular pepperoni is a good way to balance your calorie intake while studying.

Broccoli and Rice Casserole
Cheesy and good like the original...

Ingredients:
- 1/4 cup white rice
- 1/2 cup **chicken stock**, or water
- 1/2 cup broccoli flowerets, fresh or frozen
- 5 oz. can **chicken**, drained; or **seasoned tofu**
- 1/2 cup **rice, soy, almond or dairy milk**
- 2 oz. **soy cheese** or dairy cheese

Rice Cooker Directions:
Combine rice and stock in the rice cooker. Turn on and when it clicks over to warm, add the milk, chicken, broccoli and cheese. Stir. Turn back onto high and cook until the cheese melts. Makes 2 portions.

Nutrition Information...
Calories: 345   Protein: 22 g   Carbs: 29 g   Fat: 14 g

*C*reative Cooking...
Instead of chicken, try ham, tofu, or turkey.
Add vegetables such as diced red pepper, peas, mushrooms, etc.
Spice it up with hot sauce or crushed red pepper.
Instead of white rice, use brown rice and 1/2 cup more water.
Top with sliced toasted almonds.

*S*hopping Tip...
Get just the amount of broccoli and other vegetables you want from the salad bar of your grocery store.

Hearty Meals

This way to hungry-ville

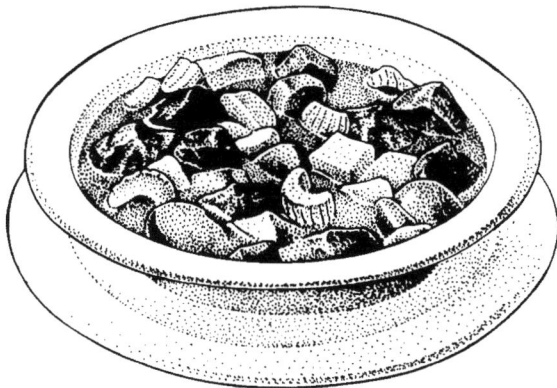

Southwest Corn and Bean Soup

An easy soup for quick suppers

Ingredients:

- 1 -8 oz. can **corn** with liquid
- 1 -14 oz. can **kidney beans**, undrained
- 1 -14 oz. can **diced tomatoes**
- 1 -8 oz. can **tomato sauce**
- 1 small onion, diced
- 2 Tbsp. **taco seasoning mix**
- 3 oz. **soy cheese**, or dairy American cheese

Rice Cooker or Stovetop Directions:

Combine all ingredients in a large saucepan or rice cooker. Heat on medium stirring occasionally until the soup is hot and bubbly. Top with corn chips if desired. Makes 2 portions.

Microwave Directions:

Combine all ingredients in a 2 quart microwave container. Cover with vent and cook on high for 4 minutes. Stir and cook in 30 second intervals until hot. Makes 2 portions.

Nutrition Information:
Calories: 259   Protein: 11 g   Carbs: 44 g   Fat: 5 g

Note: Items listed in **bold** in the recipes have a higher incidence of containing gluten – it's a **reminder** to always check the label or directly with the manufacturer.

Taco Soup

Everything tacos – top with sour cream or hot peppers

Ingredients:

- ♦ 1/2 lb. ground beef, ground turkey or ground chicken
- ♦ ½ -14 oz. can corn, drained
- ♦ 1 -14 oz. can **diced tomatoes** with green chilies
- ♦ 1 cup **kidney beans**, drained
- ♦ 1 cup water
- ♦ 1 cup salsa
- ♦ 2 Tbsp. **taco seasoning mix**
- ♦ 1 **corn tortilla**, cut in strips

Recipe Directions:

In a skillet or rice cooker, brown ground beef until no longer pink. Drain the fat and add the taco seasoning. Add the rest of the ingredients, stirring well. Bring to a boil, and then reduce the heat to a simmer (low heat). Cook for 8-12 minutes. Makes 2 portions.

Nutrition Information:

Calories: 525   Protein: 31 g   Carbs: 59 g   Fat: 18 g

Cheeseburger Chowder

Meat and potatoes in one pot

Ingredients:
- ♦ 1/2 lb. ground beef (or turkey, chicken, seasoned tofu)
- ♦ 1 Tbsp. **taco seasoning mix**
- ♦ 1 cup **rice, soy, almond or dairy milk**
- ♦ 1 cup frozen **hash brown potatoes,** or shredded fresh
  potato
- ♦ 2 oz. **soy cheese** or dairy cheese

Rice Cooker or Stovetop Directions:
In a 2-quart saucepan or rice cooker, brown the hamburger until no longer pink. Drain the fat from the meat. Add the taco seasoning and mix well. Add the rest of the ingredients and cook over medium heat until the cheese has melted, about 10-15 minutes. Makes 2 portions.

Microwave Directions:
In a 2-quart microwave container, brown the hamburger until no longer pink, cooking and stirring in 1 minute intervals. Drain the fat from the meat. Add the taco seasoning and mix well. Add the rest of the ingredients and continue cooking until the cheese has melted. Let rest for 3-4 minutes. Makes 2 portions.

Nutrition Information:
Calories: 490   Protein: 27 g   Carbs: 29 g   Fat: 27 g

● ● ● ● ● ● ● ● ● ● ● ● ● ●

Northwest Chili

A vegan chili that is a full meal

Ingredients:

- ◆ 1- 8 fl oz. can **tomato juice**
- ◆ 1 cup water
- ◆ 1/4 cup lentils, washed
- ◆ 1 potato, diced
- ◆ 6 baby carrots, sliced
- ◆ 1 -14 oz. can **garbanzo beans** (chickpeas), drained
- ◆ 1 tsp. minced onion
- ◆ 1 tsp. **chili powder**, or more to taste
- ◆ 1 cube (or 1 tsp.) **vegetable bouillon**

Recipe Directions:

Cut the potato into small pieces (dice). Cut each baby carrot into 5 pieces. In a large saucepan or rice cooker, combine the tomato juice, water, diced potato, carrots and lentils. When the mixture starts to boil, turn the heat to medium low and simmer for 10 minutes. Stir occasionally. Add the drained garbanzo beans, bouillon cube and spices. Simmer on low until the lentils and potatoes are tender, about 10 more minutes. Serve as is or with steamed rice. Makes 2 portions.

Microwave Directions:

Cut the potato into small pieces (dice). Cut each baby carrot into 5 pieces. In a 2-quart microwave safe container, combine the tomato juice, water, diced potato, carrots and lentils. Loosely cover and cook on high for 6 minutes. Add the drained garbanzo beans, bouillon cube and spices. Stir well and cook until the potatoes and lentils are tender, about 6 more minutes. Allow to rest 5 minutes. Serve as is or with steamed rice.

Nutrition Information:
Calories: 375   Protein: 20 g   Carbs: 66 g   Fat: 4 g

Tex-i-can Chili

A spicy version of chili with little effort

Ingredients:

- 4 oz. **deli roast beef**, cut into ½" slices and then diced
- 1 -14 oz. can **diced tomatoes** w/green pepper & onion
- 1/4 cup salsa, hot
- 1 -15 oz. can dark **red kidney beans**, drained
- 2 tsp. **chili powder**
- 1/2 tsp. garlic powder
- 1 tsp. corn or potato starch

Recipe Directions:

In a medium saucepan or rice cooker, combine the diced tomatoes and the potato starch. Stir until the starch is dissolved. Add the drained kidney beans, salsa and spices. Heat on medium. Cut the cooked roast beef into small pieces. Add the meat when the chili is starting to bubble. Cook for 5-8 minutes more on simmer (low), stirring occasionally. Makes 2 portions.

Microwave Directions:

In a 2 quart microwave container, combine the diced tomatoes and the potato starch. Stir until the starch is dissolved. Add the drained kidney beans, salsa and spices. Microwave loosely covered for 4-6 minutes. Meanwhile, cut the cooked roast beef into small pieces. Add the meat to the chili, stir, and cook for 2-3 more minutes), stirring occasionally. Allow to rest for 5 minutes. Makes 2 portions.

C reative Cooking...
Add a small can of well-drained corn; fresh peppers and onions at the start of cooking; or top with crumbled corn chips for crunch. You can also replace the cooked beef with diced turkey, canned chicken, or sliced cooked sausages.

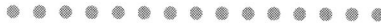

Corn Chowder

Corn, cheese, and potatoes - what could be better?

Ingredients:

- ◆ 1 -8 oz. can **creamed corn**
- ◆ 1/2 cup water
- ◆ 1 cube (or teaspoon) **chicken or vegetable bouillon**
- ◆ 1/4 cup **rice, soy, almond, or dairy milk**
- ◆ 1 small potato, diced in small pieces
- ◆ 1 tsp. onion flakes, dehydrated
- ◆ 2 oz. **soy cheese** or substitute

Rice Cooker Directions:

Combine all ingredients in rice cooker. Mix well and turn on. Cook for 16-20 minutes until the potatoes are tender. Makes 2 portions.

Stovetop Directions:

Combine all ingredients in a medium saucepan. Turn on medium. Cook for 16-20 minutes, stirring occasionally, until the potatoes are tender.

Microwave Directions:

Combine all ingredients in a 2 quart microwavable container. Mix well, cover loosely, and microwave on high for 7 minutes. Stir and continue cooking until the potatoes are tender, about 2-3 more minutes. Soup will be very hot - cool slightly before tasting. Makes 2 portions.

Nutrition Information...
Calories: 248   Protein: 9 g   Carbs: 46 g   Fat: 9 g

Creative Cooking...
Add diced bacon or ham, diced green or red peppers, broccoli, or peas, or hot sauce.

Curried Cheese Chowder

A taste of India in a warm and thick soup...

Ingredients:
- 1 cup cauliflower, cut into small pieces
- 1/2 small red pepper, diced
- 1 potato, cut into small pieces
- 1 tsp. **chicken or vegetable bouillon**
- 1 cup water
- 1 tsp. onion flakes, dehydrated
- 1/2 tsp. **curry powder**
- 1/4 cup **rice, soy, almond, or dairy milk**
- 2 oz. meltable **soy cheese** or dairy cheese

Rice Cooker Directions:
Combine chicken stock, cauliflower, pepper, potato, onion flakes, and curry powder. Turn on and cook for 15 minutes. Add the soy cheese and rice milk (or substitute). Continue to cook for 5 more minutes and turn to warm. Makes 2 portions.

Microwave Directions:
Combine chicken stock, cauliflower, pepper, potato, onion flakes, and curry powder in a 2 quart microwavable container. Cover loosely, and cook on high for 8 minutes. Add the soy cheese and rice milk (or substitute). Continue to cook for 3-5 more minutes. Allow to cool slightly before serving. Makes 2 portions.

Nutrition Information...
Calories: 219   Protein: 10 g   Carbs: 37g   Fat: 5 g

*C*reative Cooking...
Add green peas, chick peas, or other vegetables at the same time as the cheese and milk.
Add cooked, diced chicken, turkey, or bacon.
Add coconut milk instead of rice milk.

Chicken Noodle Soup
Just the best comfort food of all time...

Ingredients:
- ♦ 1 cup water
- ♦ 1 tsp. **chicken bouillon**
- ♦ 1 -5 oz. can chicken with broth
- ♦ 1/4 cup **rice noodles** or rice spaghetti noodles, broken into 1" pieces
- ♦ 1 tsp. minced onion
- ♦ 1/4 tsp. **all purpose seasoning**

Rice Cooker Directions:
Combine stock, canned chicken with broth, onion and spices. Turn cooker on high. When the soup boils (bubbles), add the noodles (break into small pieces if desired). Stir and cook for 5 minutes. Turn to warm and cover for 5 minutes. Makes 2 portions.

Microwave Directions:
Combine stock, canned chicken with broth, onion and spices in a 2 quart microwave container. Cover loosely. Cook for 4 minutes on high. Add the noodles (break into small pieces if desired). Stir and cook for 4 minutes more. Allow to sit for 2 minutes. Makes 2 portions.

Nutrition Information...
Calories: 149   Protein: 17 g   Carbs: 6 g   Fat: 6 g

Creative Cooking...
Add fresh diced onion, pepper, celery, or carrot to the broth at the start.
Add leftover cooked rice or pasta instead of noodles.

Hot and Sour Soup

Better than takeout because it's gluten free

Ingredients:

- ♦ 2 tsp. cornstarch or potato starch
- ♦ 1 1/2 cups **chicken or vegetable stock**
- ♦ 1 Tbsp. **soy sauce or tamari**
- ♦ 1/2 tsp. **Thai chili sauce**
- ♦ 1/4 packet sugar, granulated (1/4 tsp. sugar)
- ♦ 1/2 cup **oriental vegetables**, fresh or frozen
- ♦ 1/4 block **tofu**, extra firm, cut into small strips (1" long x 1/2" wide)
- ♦ 2 Tbsp. brown rice vinegar
- ♦ 1/4 tsp. toasted sesame oil
- ♦ 1 large egg, beaten

Rice Cooker Directions:

Mix cornstarch with the stock in the rice cooker or saucepan. Turn on cooker (stovetop – medium heat) and add the soy sauce, chili sauce, sugar, and vegetables. Heat until the vegetables are almost cooked, about 8-10 minutes. Add the vinegar and sesame oil. Crack the egg into a small bowl and beat until smooth with a fork. Stir the soup with the fork, and at the same time, drizzle the egg into the soup while it is boiling. Serve immediately.

Nutrition Information...
Calories: 143   Protein: 13 g   Carbs: 8 g   Fat: 5 g

S hopping Tip...

Make sure you purchase gluten free oriental sauces. Even tofu can contain wheat, so check those labels!
Shop the salad bar at the grocery store for your vegetables. You can find baby corn, broccoli, water chestnuts, bean sprouts, snow peas, carrots, and more for your soup.

• • • • • • • • • • • • • •

Vegetarian Chili

A thick and hearty chili as hot as you want it...

Ingredients:

♦ 1 -14 oz. can **stewed tomato**, Mexican recipe
♦ 1 -8 oz. can **tomato sauce**
♦ 1 -14 oz. can **black beans**, drained
♦ 1 -8 oz. can **corn**, drained
♦ 1/2 small onion, diced
♦ 1 tsp. **chili powder**
♦ 1/2 tsp. cumin, ground
♦ 1/2 tsp. black pepper, ground

Rice Cooker Directions:

Combine all ingredients and cook for 15-22 minutes. Makes 2 large portions.

Microwave Directions:

Combine all ingredients in a 2-quart microwave container loosely covered. Cook on high for 8 minutes, stir, and continue to cook in 30 second intervals until bubbly hot. Allow to cool slightly before eating. Makes 2 large portions.

Nutrition Information...
Calories: 383   Protein: 16 g   Carbs: 76 g   Fat: 2 g

C reative Cooking...
Add tofu, or fresh vegetables like mushrooms, green beans, or peppers.
Add soy (or dairy) sour cream or crunchy corn chips to top off the chili.
Add more chili powder and cumin to taste. Spice up the heat with red pepper or hot sauce.

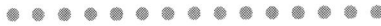
Minestrone

Don't let the number of ingredients stop you – this is easy!

Ingredients:

- 1 cup carrot, sliced
- 1 cup celery, sliced
- 1 small zucchini, diced
- 1 small green pepper, diced
- 1 small onion, diced
- 1 Tbsp. olive oil
- 1 -14 oz can **cannellini beans**, drained
- 1 cube **bouillon, beef or vegetable**
- 1 cup water
- 1 -14 oz. can **diced chili** tomatoes
- 3 oz. brown rice spiral or elbow pasta (about 1 cup)
- 1 tsp. basil, dried

Rice Cooker or Stovetop Directions:

In a rice cooker or 2 quart pan heat the olive oil. Add the carrots, celery, zucchini, pepper, and onion. Cook for 3-4 minutes, or until vegetables start to soften. Stir in the remaining ingredients. Cover and cook (on medium) for 15-20 minutes. Sprinkle with Parmesan cheese if desired. Makes 4 portions.

Microwave Directions:

In a 2 quart microwave safe container, combine the carrots, celery, zucchini, pepper, and onion. Drizzle with oil: toss to coat. Cover and microwave on high for 5 minutes. Stir in the remaining ingredients. Cover and cook on high for 15 minutes. Allow to rest 5 minutes before eating. Sprinkle with Parmesan cheese if desired. Makes 4 portions.

Nutrition Information:
Calories: 215   Protein: 7 g   Carbs: 38 g   Fat: 4 g

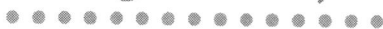

Taco Meat
- Beef, Chicken, Turkey or Tofu

Ingredients:
- ♦ 1/2 lb raw ground beef, ground turkey, ground chicken, or crumbled extra firm tofu
- ♦ 1 -8 oz. can **tomato sauce**
- ♦ 1 Tbsp. **taco seasoning mix**

Rice Cooker Directions:
Put the ground beef in the rice cooker and turn on. Stir often until meat is cooked (no red showing). Return to the heat - turn on high. Add the tomato sauce and the taco seasoning. Cook for 7-10 minutes. Serves 3

Microwave Directions:
Break up ground meat in a 2 quart microwave safe container. Cook on high for 2-3 minutes. Stir and microwave until the meat is cooked. Drain off the fat into a container - discard appropriately. Add tomato sauce and seasoning. Cook for an additional 3-5 minutes.

Nutrition Information...
Calories: 191   Protein: 15 g   Carbs: 6 g   Fat: 11 g

C *reative Cooking......*
Add diced onion, peppers, jalapeno peppers, corn kernels, black beans, etc.
Make tacos, burrito wraps, taco salad, top a baked potato, or layer with refried beans and salsa for a dip.

Teriyaki Chicken
Sweet and tangy, a great meal...

Ingredients:
- ◆ 1 chicken breast, boneless, raw (about 4-5 oz.)
- ◆ 2 Tbsp. **soy sauce or tamari**
- ◆ 1 tsp. lemon juice or rice vinegar
- ◆ 1 packet sugar
- ◆ 1/4 tsp. garlic powder

Mix the soy sauce, sugar, lemon juice, and garlic together in a bowl. Marinate the raw chicken breast in the teriyaki sauce for at least one hour and up to 24 hours under refrigeration.

Rice Cooker Directions:
Put the marinated chicken and sauce into the rice cooker. Turn on and cover. Check after 5-6 minutes and turn chicken over. Cook until center reaches 165° degrees F. on a meat thermometer. Add a little water if pan goes dry before chicken is cooked.

Microwave Directions:
Cover the chicken in a microwave safe bowl or plate. Cook 3 minutes and turn over to cook 2-3 minutes more. Allow to rest for 1 minute. Check that the chicken reaches 165° degrees F. in the center on a meat thermometer.

Nutrition Information...
Calories: 204   Protein: 37 g   Carbs: 7 g   Fat: 2 g

C reative Cooking...
Add a drop of sesame oil, or sesame seeds in the marinade. Serve with rice and steamed vegetables.

S hopping Tip...
Make more than one and have a cold sliced chicken salad or stir fry the next day.

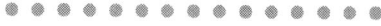

Jammed Ham

*Shopping Tip- Ask for one 1/2" thick slice of ham
from the deli counter.*

Ingredients:
- ♦ 1 slice **ham steak**
- ♦ 1 Tbsp. jam or jelly (like apricot, cherry, or orange marmalade)
- ♦ 1 -4 oz. fruit cup or mandarin orange cup

Recipe Directions:
In a small skillet or rice cooker, drain the liquid from the fruit cup into the pan. Heat until steaming. Add the ham steak and spread the fruit over the top of the ham. Drizzle the jam over the ham. Cook until the liquid evaporates. Makes 1 portion.

Nutrition Information:
Calories: 180   Protein: 11 g   Carbs: 27 g   Fat: 2 g

C ooking Tip...
Cook frozen or fresh vegetables along side the ham steak.

Tamari Tofu
Caramelized and crispy

Ingredients:

- ♦ 8 oz. **tofu**, firm
- ♦ 2 tsp. **soy sauce or tamari**
- ♦ 1 tsp. orange juice
- ♦ 1/4 tsp. toasted sesame oil
- ♦ 1 tsp. honey
- ♦ 1/4 tsp. garlic powder
- ♦ 1/2 tsp. canola oil

Grill Machine or Stovetop Directions:

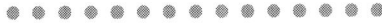

Preheat a grill machine, or heat a small skillet on medium. Use paper towels to press water out of tofu and cut into 1/4 inch slices. Combine remaining ingredients, except oil, in a shallow bowl. Dip tofu slices into sauce. Brush oil or cooking spray oil over both grilling surfaces or in the skillet. Arrange tofu on hot grill. Close cover and cook about 4 minutes, or until golden. If using a skillet, check bottoms for golden brown color, and turn over. Cook until golden on other side. Add vegetable slices to the grill or skillet to complement your meal.

Nutrition Information...
Calories: 248   Protein: 20 g   Carbs: 10g   Fat: 14g

* * * * * * * * * * * * * *

Garlic Shrimp
A special dinner

Ingredients:
- ♦ 2 Tbsp. butter or olive oil
- ♦ 1 tsp. garlic powder or minced fresh garlic
- ♦ 4 oz. shrimp, raw and deveined, medium size
- ♦ 1/2 tsp. basil
- ♦ 2 tsp. grated **non-dairy or dairy Parmesan cheese**

Recipe Directions:
In a 1-quart microwave container, melt the butter or margarine with the garlic and basil - about 40-60 seconds. Add the shrimp and coat with the butter. Cook on 70% power for 1 to 1 1/2 minutes. Shrimp should be firm and opaque. Stir in Parmesan cheese.

The shrimp can be served as a main meal over cooked rice, or with toothpicks for a special snack.

Nutrition Information:
Calories: 350   Protein: 25 g   Carbs: 4 g   Fat: 26 g

Popcorn Chicken

Little breaded chicken poppers go great with dips.
Reheat in a microwave if there are extras!

Ingredients:

- 1/3 cup **mayonnaise**
- 2 Tbsp. **Dijon mustard**
- 1 Tbsp. lemon juice or rice vinegar
- 1/2 tsp. **hot pepper sauce**
- 1 cup GF **bread crumbs**; or crushed GF **rice cereal**
- 1 tsp. salt
- 1 tsp. **all purpose seasoning blend**
- 1 lb. chicken breast, cut into 1" cubes

Recipe Directions:

Cut the chicken breast into 1" pieces. Preheat the oven, or toaster oven, to 450° degrees F. Line the baking sheet with aluminum foil and lightly grease with vegetable oil.

Combine the mayonnaise, mustard, juice, and hot sauce in a medium bowl. Add the chicken pieces and toss to cover with the mixture. In a separate plate, or piece of wax paper, combine the crumbs, salt and seasoning. Mix well with a fork. Drop pieces of chicken into the breading and roll around until covered. Put on the baking sheet, allowing a little space between pieces. Continue breading all the chicken.

Put in the oven and bake for 10 minutes. Flip the pieces over and bake until all sides are brown and the chicken is done inside, about 6-8 minutes more. Serve with your favorite dip or dressing. Makes 4 portions.

Nutrition Information:
Calories: 318   Protein: 22 g   Carbs: 13g   Fat: 19 g

Teriyaki Chicken Wings

Spicy with a hint of sweetness

Ingredients:
♦ 12 wings chicken wings, raw
♦ 1/4 cup **soy sauce or tamari**
♦ 2 Tbsp. brown sugar
♦ 1 tsp. garlic powder
♦ 1 tsp. **Thai chili sauce**

Recipe Directions:
Combine all ingredients in a large zip bag. Marinate for at least 2 hours and up to 24 hours.

Preheat the toaster oven or regular oven to 425° degrees F. Cover a baking sheet with aluminum foil and lightly oil the surface. Place the wings on the baking sheet with space around them. Bake for 10 minutes and turn over. Continue baking until skin is crispy and the joints move easily. Makes 2 portions

Nutrition Information:
Calories: 303   Protein: 42 g   Carbs: 15 g   Fat: 6 g

C reative Cooking...
After cooking, drizzle with honey and sprinkle with sesame seeds if desired.

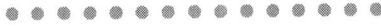

Breaded Chicken Fingers

A little kitchen work makes a great meal

Ingredients:

- ◆ 1 lb chicken tenderloins, raw;
  or raw boneless chicken breast cut into ½" strips
- ◆ 1 cup gluten free flour mix
- ◆ 1 tsp. salt, or **seasoning blend** of choice
- ◆ 1/2 tsp. black pepper
- ◆ 1/4 tsp. baking powder
- ◆ ¼ tsp. Xanthan gum
- ◆ 1 large egg, beaten with 1 Tbsp. water
- ◆ GF **cooking oil spray**

Recipe Directions:

Makes 4 portions. Preheat the toaster oven to 425° degrees F. Line a baking sheet with aluminum foil or a silicone liner. Wash and dry the chicken meat. In a small, flat bowl, beat the egg and water with a fork. In a flat plate, combine the gluten free flour, seasonings, baking powder and Xanthan gum. Add other spices at this time if desired. Mix with a fork until evenly combined.

Dip each chicken piece into the flour mixture, then into the egg, and back into the flour mixture. Lay on the baking sheet. Keep pieces separate (not touching). Continue with all the tenders. Spray lightly with a cooking oil spray.

Bake immediately for 12-14 minutes. Turn over, lightly spray again with cooking oil spray, and bake for 5-8 minutes more.

Nutrition Information:
Calories: 256   Protein: 24 g   Carbs: 33 g   Fat: 2 g

S ubstitutions...
If you have a gluten free baking or pancake mix, you can use 1 cup and leave out the 3-flour mix, salt, Xanthan gum, and baking powder.

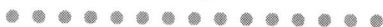

College Drums
Easy chicken drumsticks...

Ingredients:
- ♦ 1 lb. chicken drumsticks
- ♦ 3 Tbsp. **soy sauce or tamari**
- ♦ 1/2 cup ketchup
- ♦ 3 Tbsp. orange juice
- ♦ 1/2 tsp. garlic powder

Rice Cooker Directions:
In the rice cooker, combine the soy sauce or tamari, ketchup, orange juice, and garlic. Mix well. Add the drumsticks and turn to coat in the sauce. Turn the rice cooker on and simmer until the drumsticks are thoroughly cooked (165°F. on a food thermometer) - about 20-25 minutes. Turn the rice cooker to warm until you are ready to serve the drums.

Microwave Directions:
In a 2 quart microwavable container, combine the soy sauce or tamari, ketchup, orange juice, and garlic. Mix well. Add the drumsticks and turn to coat in the sauce. Cook on high for 8 minutes. Stir and continue to cook in 30 second intervals until the drumsticks are thoroughly cooked (165°F. on a food thermometer). Let rest 5 minutes.

Nutrition Information...
Calories: 372   Protein: 40g   Carbs: 42 g   Fat: 3 g

C reative Cooking......
You can substitute one pound chicken thighs, wings or boneless chicken breast in this recipe. Add hot sauce to taste. If you would like to reduce the fat in this dish, take the skin off the chicken before cooking.

S hopping Tip...
You can buy chicken drumsticks or thighs for less money than most other pieces of the chicken.

Chicken and Waffles

The famous diner dish, only gluten free

Ingredients:

- ◆ 1/3 cup **cooked chicken** (about 1- 5oz. canned chicken, drained)
- ◆ 2 oz. **cream cheese** alternative, or dairy cream cheese
- ◆ 1/3 cup **chicken stock** (or one **bouillon** cube dissolved in 1/3 cup water)
- ◆ 1 stalk celery, diced
- ◆ 3 baby carrots, sliced
- ◆ ¼ tsp. **all purpose seasoning blend**
- ◆ 1 gluten free waffle

Rice Cooker Directions:

Combine the celery, carrot, chicken stock (or water and bouillon cube), cream cheese in the rice cooker and turn on high setting. Once the mixture comes to a boil, stir often until smooth. Add the chicken meat and seasonings. Heat till bubbly. Toast the waffle and pour the chicken mixture over the top.

Stovetop Directions:

Combine the celery, carrot, chicken stock (or water and bouillon cube), cream cheese in a 1-quart saucepan and put on medium heat. Once the mixture comes to a boil, stir often until smooth and turn to medium low heat. Add the cooked chicken meat and seasonings. Heat until bubbly. Toast the waffle and pour the chicken mixture over the top.

Microwave Directions:

Combine the celery, carrot, chicken stock (or water and bouillon cube), cream cheese in a 1-quart microwave safe container. Cook on high, covered and vented, for 2 minutes. Stir and heat in 15 second intervals until the sauce can be stirred smooth. Add the chicken meat and seasonings. Heat 30-60 seconds more. Toast the waffle and pour the chicken mixture over the top.

Nutrition Information...
Calories: 437   Protein: 29 g   Carbs: 21 g   Fat: 26 g

Ham and Cheese Potato Skins

A restaurant favorite that you can enjoy in your dorm room

Ingredients:

- 1 small baked potato
- 2 Tbsp. **rice, soy, almond, or dairy milk**
- 2 Tbsp. **sour cream alternative**, or dairy sour cream
- 1 tsp. **prepared mustard**
- 2 oz. **ham**, diced; or ¼ cup **seasoned tofu**
- 1 slice **soy cheese**, or dairy American cheese

Recipe Directions:

Microwave a baked potato. Allow to cool 10 minutes or more. Cut the potato in half lengthwise and using a spoon, scoop out the potato into a small bowl. Using a fork, mash the potato with the milk, sour cream, and mustard until well combined. Stir in the ham (or tofu) and cheese. Mound the mixture back into the potato skin shells. Microwave on high for 2 - 3 minutes. Makes 1 portion.

Nutrition Information:
Calories: 448   Protein: 36 g   Carbs: 27 g   Fat: 22 g

Hamburger Gravy

*This is real comfort food, with all the flavor
of beef stroganoff*

Ingredients:

- ♦ 1/2 lb. ground beef
- ♦ 1/2 cup water
- ♦ 1 cube (or 1 teaspoon) **beef bouillon**
- ♦ 1/4 cup **sour cream alternative,** or dairy sour cream

Stovetop Instructions:

Crumble hamburger into saucepan and stir until brown; drain. Add water, bouillon, and pepper to taste. Cook 5 minutes, stirring occasionally. Stir in sour cream and heat for an additional minute. Serve over toast, rice or noodles. Makes 2 portions.

Microwave Instructions:

Break up ground beef in a 2 quart microwave container. Cook for 2-3 minutes on high until beef is browned, and drain off the fat. Add the water and bouillon, stir, cover loosely and cook for 2-3 minutes until hot all the way through. Stir in sour cream and heat for an additional minute. Serve over toast, rice or noodles. Makes 2 portions.

Nutrition Information...
Calories: 288   Protein: 23 g   Carbs: 9 g   Fat: 18 g

Easy Beef Chili

Can't get more basic than this – make a big batch for exams

Ingredients:

- 1/2 lb. lean ground beef; OR ground turkey or chicken
- 1- 14 oz. can **red kidney beans**, drained well
- 1- 14 oz. can **diced tomatoes**
- 1- 8 oz. can **tomato sauce**
- 1 Tbsp. minced onion (dried spice), or 2 Tbsp. fresh diced onion
- 2 tsp. **chili powder,** or more to taste
- 1/2 tsp. cumin, ground
- 1/2 tsp. black pepper, or ¼ tsp red pepper flakes
- ¼ tsp. salt

Rice Cooker Directions:

Break up ground beef in rice cooker. Drain the fat. Add all other ingredients. Turn to high and cook for 20 minutes stirring once in a while. Makes 4 portions.

Stovetop Directions:

Break up ground beef in a large saucepan on medium heat. Cook until browned and drain the fat. Add all of the other ingredients. Turn to medium low and cook for 20 minutes stirring once in a while. Makes 4 portions.

Microwave Directions:

Break up ground beef in a 2 quart microwave container. Cook for 2-3 minutes on high until beef is browned, and drain off the fat. Add the rest of ingredients, stir, cover loosely and cook for 6-10 minutes until hot all the way through. Allow to cool slightly before eating. Makes 4 portions.

Nutrition Information...
Calories: 226   Protein: 18 g   Carbs: 25 g   Fat: 6 g

Rice Cooker, Microwave
Vegan Friendly
● ● ● ● ● ● ● ● ● ● ● ● ● ● ● ●

Barbequed Beans with Sausage
Hearty and filling for fall weather

Ingredients:
- 1 -14 oz. can **black beans**, drained well
- 1/2 cup **barbeque sauce**
- 4 oz. smoked **Italian sausage** or **bratwurst**, fully cooked; or **vegan substitute**
- 1/4 cup water

Rice Cooker Directions:
Cut the smoked sausage into "coins" about 1/4" thick. Drain the black beans. Put all ingredients in the rice cooker and turn on high. Cook for 10-15 minutes or until hot and slightly thick.

Microwave Directions:
Cut the smoked sausage into "coins" about 1/4" thick. Drain the black beans. Put all ingredients (except the water) in a 2 quart microwave container, loosely cover, and cook for 6-8 minutes or until hot and slightly thick. You will not need the extra water in the microwave. Very Hot - allow to cool before eating.

Nutrition Information...
Calories: 405   Protein: 18 g   Carbs: 65 g   Fat: 6 g

C reative Cooking...
 Add onions and peppers, diced or sliced
 Use canned pinto beans instead of black beans and salsa instead of barbeque sauce for Mexican Beans.
Add soy chorizo instead of meat sausage for a vegan meal.

Sides

Flying solo or in tandem with a meal - easy fixin's

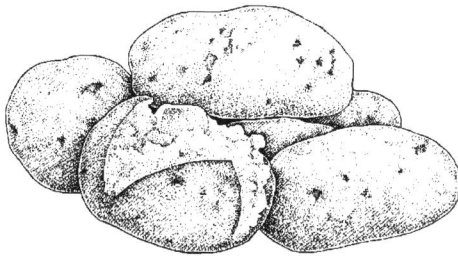

Honey Mustard Roast Potatoes

*Leave the fast food French Fries alone –
real roast potatoes in a flash*

Ingredients:

♦ 2 medium red potatoes (or 6 small)
♦ 1 tsp. cooking oil
♦ 1/2 tsp. onion powder
♦ 1/2 tsp. honey
♦ 1/2 tsp. **mustard, prepared**
♦ 1/4 tsp. salt

Recipe Directions:

Heat the toaster oven, or regular oven to 400° degrees F. Cover a baking sheet with aluminum foil.

Cut the potatoes into 3/4" cubes. In a bowl, mix the oil, mustard, honey and seasonings. Add the potato cubes and stir until the potatoes are coated with the seasonings. Pour onto the baking sheet and bake for 20 to 30 minutes, stirring once. Bake until the potatoes can be pierced easily with a fork.

Nutrition Information:
Calories: 301   Protein: 7 g   Carbs: 58 g   Fat: 5 g

Note: Items listed in **bold** in the recipes have a higher incidence of containing gluten – it's a ***reminder*** to always check the label or directly with the manufacturer.

• • • • • • • • • • • • • • • •

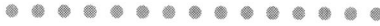

Orange Infused Dhal

An Asian dish made easy for college living

Ingredients:

♦ 2/3 cup red lentils
♦ 1/2 cup water
♦ 1/2 cup orange juice
♦ 1 Tbsp. vegetable oil
♦ 1/2 small onion, diced
♦ 1/2 tsp. garlic powder
♦ 1 tsp. cumin
♦ 1 tsp. **curry powder**
♦ 1 -8 oz. can coconut milk (1 small can, or 2/3 of a larger can)

Rice Cooker or Stovetop Directions:

Combine all ingredients in the rice cooker *or* medium pot on stove. Cook until the lentils are tender and the sauce is thick. Manually flip the rice cooker switch to keep warm.

Microwave Directions:

In a 2-quart microwave safe container, combine the lentils, water and orange juice. Cook on high for 10 minutes, covered and vented. In a separate bowl, combine the oil, spices, and onion. Microwave on high, covered and vented for 2 minutes. Stir the onion mixture and coconut milk into the lentils. Cook on high for and additional 4 minutes.

Mix well and serve over rice or as a dip with vegetables or rice crackers. Makes 2 portions.

Nutrition Information:
Calories: 238   Protein: 8 g   Carbs: 22 g   Fat: 15 g

Polenta for One
When one portion is just what you want

Ingredients:
- ♦ 1 cup water
- ♦ 1/4 cup cornmeal, or polenta
- ♦ 1 tsp. **margarine,** butter, or olive oil
- ♦ 1/8 tsp. salt
- ♦ 1 Tbsp. **Parmesan substitute** or dairy Parmesan

Microwave Instructions:
In a 1-quart glass measuring cup or bowl, stir together the water, polenta, salt, and butter. Cook, uncovered, in a microwave oven at full power, stirring once after 3 minutes, until polenta is tender and liquid is absorbed, about 7 to 8 minutes total. Spoon polenta onto plate and sprinkle with cheese.

Nutrition Information...
Calories: 156   Protein: 6 g   Carbs: 23 g   Fat: 6 g

Polenta Fries

Excellent with a little warm marinara sauce to dip

Ingredients:

- ♦ 1/3 cup cornmeal or polenta
- ♦ 1/2 cup **rice, soy, almond or dairy milk**
- ♦ 1/2 cup water
- ♦ 1/4 tsp. salt
- ♦ 1/8 cup **non-dairy or dairy Parmesan**
- ♦ 1 Tbsp. vegetable oil

Recipe Directions:

Heat the milk, water and salt in a saucepan, rice cooker, or microwave until hot. Sprinkle cornmeal over the top as you stir it in. Continue cooking and stirring until the mixture becomes very thick. Stir in the cheese. Immediately pour out onto a baking sheet and using the back of a spoon, spread the polenta to 1/2" thick. Chill for at least 2 hours or overnight.

Cut the polenta into long strips about 1/2" wide, and then across the strips in 2" intervals. This will make strips the size of potato fries. Using a pancake turner, loosen the polenta strips and put them into a large bowl. Drizzle the oil over the fries, season with salt, pepper, or herb mixture, and toss lightly so not to break them up.

Heat a toaster oven or regular oven to 450° degrees F. Cover a baking sheet with aluminum foil and lightly oil. Spread out the polenta fries evenly on the pan. Bake for 10 minutes and using a turner, flip the fries. Continue baking for 10 minutes or until the fries are golden brown. Makes 2 portions.

Nutrition Information:
Calories: 185   Protein: 6 g   Carbs: 23 g   Fat: 9 g

Sweet Potato and Apple Casserole
Vegetables with the taste of dessert

Ingredients:
- ♦ 1 medium sweet potato, baked
- ♦ 1/3 cup **apple pie filling**

Recipe Directions:
Bake or microwave the sweet potato. Scoop out the potato into a microwave safe 2-cup container. Mix in the pie filling. Sprinkle with cinnamon if desired. Microwave for 2-3 minutes until hot. Makes 1 portion.

Nutrition Information:
Calories: 193   Protein: 2 g   Carbs: 46 g   Fat: 0.17 g

Spiced Zucchini

A cool way to eat your vegetables hot

Ingredients:
- 1 small zucchini
- 1 tsp. **chili powder**, or Creole seasoning
- 1 tsp. canola oil
- 1/4 tsp. salt
- 1/2 tsp. granulated sugar or other sweetener

Recipe Directions:
Preheat toaster oven to 425° degrees F. In a bowl, toss zucchini slices with the oil until coated. Add the chili powder, salt and sugar - stir until coating is distributed. Put on a foil lined baking sheet and bake for 10-12 minutes. The squash should still be browned on the outside. Makes 1 portion.

Can also be stir-fried, adding the seasoning when the zucchini is just tender.

Nutrition Information:
Calories: 73   Protein: 1 g   Carbs: 7 g   Fat: 5 g

Ranch Hash Brown Bake

Crush corn flakes in a sealed plastic bag by rolling a full can gently over the bag

Ingredients:
- ♦ 1 cup frozen **hash brown potatoes**, or fresh shredded potato
- ♦ 1/4 cup **Ranch salad dressing**
- ♦ 2 oz. shredded **soy cheese**, or dairy cheese
- ♦ 1 Tbsp. **bacon bits**, real
- ♦ 1/4 cup **corn flake cereal**, crushed
- ♦ 1 tsp. **margarine** or substitute

Recipe Directions:
Preheat a toaster oven or regular oven to 350° degrees F. Lightly grease a small oven safe baking dish (a 4-5" diameter casserole dish works great).

In a small bowl, combine the hash browns, ranch dressing, bacon bits, and cubed or shredded cheese. Pour into the casserole dish. Top with the crushed corn flakes and dot with little pieces of margarine. Bake for 30-35 minutes or until the top is nicely browned. Makes 1 portion (or 2 as a side dish).

Nutrition Information:
Calories: 410   Protein: 7 g   Carbs: 21 g   Fat: 31 g

Roasted Maple Squash
Fall's best produce

Ingredients:
♦ 1 small Delicata squash, or small acorn squash
♦ 2 tsp. margarine
♦ 1 Tbsp. maple syrup, or pancake syrup
♦ 1/2 tsp. cinnamon, ground

Recipe Directions:
Preheat the toaster oven, or regular oven, to 400° F.

Cut the squash in half and scoop out the seeds with a spoon. Put the halves cut side up in an ovenproof baking pan. Spread the margarine over the squash. Drizzle the syrup over them and sprinkle with cinnamon. Bake for 40 minutes or until tender. May be microwaved with a vented cover - about 12 minutes. Makes 1 portion-2.

Nutrition Information:
Calories: 101   Protein: 1 g   Carbs: 17 g   Fat: 4 g

*S*hopping Tip...
Small squash or pumpkins are excellent for a filling meal with a little sweetness. Any type of small squash can be cut in half and roasted or microwaved. Be careful cutting the squash in half - start the knife tip going in and then cut slowly, keeping your hands on top of the knife. Cut on a non-slippery surface like a cutting board secured by putting a damp towel underneath. Scoop out the seeds and lay face down on a baking dish. Add a little water. Bake or microwave until soft. Add seasonings to taste.

Sweet Potato Oven Fries
Better than French fries

Ingredients:
- 1 sweet potato, well scrubbed
- 1 Tbsp. vegetable oil
- 1 tsp. **chili powder** or **all-purpose seasoning**
- 1/2 tsp. salt
- 1/2 tsp. cinnamon, ground
- 1 tsp. sugar, granulated (about one packet of sugar)

Recipe Directions:
Preheat the toaster oven to 450° degrees F. In a small bowl, mix together the cinnamon and sugar and reserve for use later.

Scrub the sweet potato under running water. Alternatively, you can peel it, but the skin is edible for this recipe. Cut the sweet potato into 1/2" thick slices and then cut each slice into 4-6 sticks so you end up with French fry size pieces. Put all the potato sticks into a bowl and toss with the oil, salt and chili powder.

On a foil-lined toaster oven sheet, spread out the sweet potatoes. Bake for 15-20 minutes, stirring once. Test for doneness by sticking a fork or knife tip into the potato - if it goes in with just a little resistance, they are done! Sprinkle with the cinnamon sugar and toss to distribute evenly. Makes 2 portions.

Nutrition Information:
Calories: 254   Protein: 2.4 g   Carbs: 31 g   Fat: 15 g

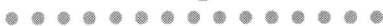

Savory Mashed Potatoes

Real mashed potatoes in 20 minutes or less...

Ingredients:

- ♦ 1 1/3 cups potato, raw, diced (about 2 medium russet potatoes or 6 small red potatoes)
- ♦ 2/3 cups **chicken stock**, or 1 tsp. **bouillon** in 2/3 c. water
- ♦ 1/2 tsp. garlic powder
- ♦ 1/4 tsp. salt (if not using bouillon)
- ♦ 2 Tbsp. **rice, soy, almond, or dairy milk**
- ♦ dash of black pepper

Rice Cooker or Stovetop Directions:

Combine all ingredients except pepper and milk in rice cooker (saucepan on stove - medium heat). Turn on and cook for 15 minutes. Remove cover and cook until the potatoes are very soft and the liquid is no more than 1/3 the volume of potatoes. Turn off cooker (remove pan from heat) and add pepper and milk. Mash potatoes right in the cooker (pan) with a non-stick masher until smooth as you like them. Potatoes should be the perfect light consistency - you can keep them warm in the cooker. Makes 2 portions.

Microwave Directions:

Combine all ingredients except pepper and milk in 2 quart microwave container. Cook covered on high for 8 minutes or until the potatoes are very soft. Mash potatoes with a potato masher. Add pepper and milk to reach the desired consistency.

Nutrition Information...
Calories: 105　　Protein: 3 g　　Carbs: 21 g　　Fat: 2 g

*C*reative Cooking...
　Add cream cheese, sour cream, butter, margarine, or chives just before mashing the potatoes.
Add diced cooked bacon, sausage or ham after mashing.
Add soy or dairy cheeses after mashing.

Microwave
Vegan
● ● ● ● ● ● ● ● ● ● ● ● ●

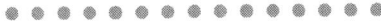

Microwave Lentils
Easy way to make lentil salad

Ingredients:
- ♦ 1 cup water
- ♦ 1/4 cup lentils

Sort through lentils and discard any debris. Rinse and drain. In a 1-quart glass measuring cup or bowl, stir together water and lentils. Cook, uncovered, in a microwave oven at full power (100 percent) until mixture boils, 3 to 4 minutes.

Cover with plastic wrap and cook at half power (50 percent) until lentils are fork tender, 12 to 14 minutes longer. Add salt to taste.

Nutrition Information...
Calories: 169   Protein: 12 g   Carbs: 28 g   Fat: 1 g

Creative Cooking......
Make an easy lentil salad for the backpack – one portion of cooked lentils from the recipe above, 1 Tbsp. of your favorite dressing, chopped carrot, celery, raisins, sunflower seeds, or whatever you have. Chill well and enjoy.

• • • • • • • • • • • • • • •

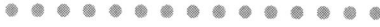

Savory Quinoa

A warm and hearty way to enjoy quinoa...

Ingredients:

♦ 1 cup water
♦ 1 cube (1 tsp.) **chicken or vegetable bouillon**
♦ 1/2 cup quinoa, washed
♦ 1/2 red pepper, chopped
♦ 1/2 cup portabella mushroom, diced; OR one can, drained
♦ 1/2 tsp. **all purpose seasoning**
♦ 1/4 tsp. granulated garlic
♦ 1/8 cup green onion, chopped (optional)

Rice Cooker Directions:

Wash quinoa in a fine sieve. Combine all ingredients except green onions in the rice cooker (or saucepan on stove). Cover and turn on to cook (medium low heat). When cooker turns off to "warm," stir in the green onion and allow the quinoa to rest for 5 minutes. On the stovetop, add the green onion when just a little water is yet to be absorbed. Cover for 5 minutes. Fluff with a fork and serve. Makes 2 portions.

Nutrition Information...
Calories: 150   Protein: 8 g   Carbs: 26 g   Fat: 2 g

Creative Cooking......

If you don't like mushrooms, add corn kernels, diced zucchini, yellow squash, or cauliflower, OR
Add golden raisins and curry powder (instead of all purpose seasoning).

Cooking Note...

Quinoa should always be washed before using as it has a bitter coating that is not tasty. Measure the amount of quinoa you want to use into a fine sieve and wash under running water. Use as you would rice in recipes.

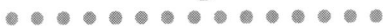

Mediterranean Polenta

Very filling as a meal with fresh vegetables

Ingredients:
- 1 cup water
- 1/3 cup cornmeal or polenta
- 3 Tbsp. fresh tomato, diced; or 1 Tbsp. dried tomatoes
- 1/4 tsp. oregano, dried
- 1/8 tsp. basil, dried
- 1/4 tsp. garlic powder

Rice Cooker Directions:
Heat 1 cup water in the rice cooker. Stir in polenta slowly. Stir as polenta cooks for about 6 to 8 minutes, add tomato and spices. Turn cooker to warm for 5 minutes.

Stovetop Directions:
Heat 1 cup water in a saucepan on medium heat. Stir in polenta slowly. Stir as polenta cooks for about 6 to 8 minutes, turning the heat down to medium low. Add spices and let rest for 5 minutes.

Nutrition Information...
Calories: 137   Protein: 3 g   Carbs: 30 g   Fat: 1 g

*C*reative *Cooking......*
Stir in crumbled feta cheese or cheese substitute, olives or other Italian vegetables. Try it for breakfast with crumbled sausage.

Curried Root Vegetables

*Hearty vegetables that will keep you full
and away from the snacks*

Ingredients:

- 1 cup **vegetable stock**,
  or 1 cube **bouillon** and 1 cup water
- 2 potatoes, diced
- 5 baby carrots, sliced
- 1/2 small onion, diced
- 1/3 cup red pepper, diced (about ¼ a small pepper)
- 1 tsp. **curry powder**

Rice Cooker Directions:

Cut up potatoes into 1/2" cubes. Cut peppers and onions to large chunks. Combine all ingredients in rice cooker and turn on. Cook until vegetables are tender and broth has reduced to a glaze – about 15-20 minutes.

Stovetop Directions:

Cut up potatoes into 1/2" cubes. Cut peppers and onions to large chunks. Combine all ingredients in a medium saucepan and turn on to medium heat. Cook until vegetables are tender and broth has reduced to a glaze – about 15-20 minutes.

Nutrient Analysis:
Calories: 321   Protein: 8 g   Carbs: 70 g   Total Fat: 1 g

*C*reative Cooking...
Add toasted nuts, bacon bits, or dried fruit like coconut, raisins, apricots or cranberries.

Sesame Green Beans

A tasty meal with rice or a side dish

Ingredients:

- 1/4 cup water
- 1 cup green beans, whole, frozen or fresh
- 1/2 tsp. toasted sesame oil
- 1/8 tsp. garlic powder
- 1 oz. cashews, raw (about 2 tablespoons)

Stovetop Directions:

In a small skillet on medium high heat, bring the water to a boil and add the green beans. Cook until the water evaporates and add the sesame oil, garlic and cashews. Stir often and cook until the beans are fork tender, about 2-3 minutes.

Nutrition Information...
Calories: 231   Protein: 6 g   Carbs: 14 g   Fat: 17 g

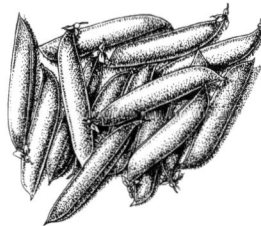

Gluten Free
Quick Reference Guide

The Gluten-Free Shopper

If you are new to eating without gluten, keep the following "do's, don'ts, and maybe's" in mind when shopping in C-stores and grocery stores. This list is gluten free only; casein free shoppers will need to check each label for dairy. All manufacturers can change food formulations at will, so check the label on everything!

Usually Gluten Free...

♦ All fresh meats, seafood, poultry, and eggs; fish canned in oil, brine, or water; cured or cooked meats like ham and bacon; many sausages and some hot dogs (always check the label).

♦ All plain fruits and vegetables (fresh, frozen, or canned); plain fruit juices; fresh and dried herbs; dried beans, peas, and lentils; olives.

♦ All plain dairy products if tolerant, including milk, cream, and butter. Sour cream, cottage cheese, and yogurt if they contain no suspect thickeners.

♦ All types of natural cheese (not processed) if tolerant, such as Cheddar, Swiss, Mozzarella, Parmesan, ricotta, goat's and sheep's milk cheeses. Check the label of processed cheeses like American or Swiss American, and cheese food snacks.

♦ Olive oil, canola oil, and other pure vegetable oils; gluten free margarine.

- All single vinegars (except malt vinegar).

- Tamari or soy sauce, if brewed solely from soybeans and marked gluten free.

- Chicken, beef, and vegetable broths, if they contain no hydrolyzed wheat protein or other source of gluten. Gluten free bouillon cubes or broth powders are available. Choose products marked gluten free.

- Jams and jellies, honey, sugar, molasses, maple syrup, pancake syrup.

- Plain chocolate (dark, milk, and white), and chocolate chips; pure cocoa powder.

- Plain nuts and nut flours; peanut butter, sunflower butter, tahini, almond butter, etc

- Tea, coffee, and pure hot chocolate and cocoa. Beware sweetened and flavored coffees, lattes and cappuccinos.

- Plain ice creams, frozen yogurt (check the labels), sorbets. Beware of mix-ins or cookie chunks containing wheat flour.

- Rice (all types: white, brown, converted, jasmine, basmati, Arborio, etc.)

- Corn (cornmeal, masa harina, grits, cornstarch, polenta, pre-cooked polenta rolls, corn tortillas, corn chips, etc.)

- Other Grains, Seeds, Roots, and Flours. Amaranth, arrowroot, buckwheat (kasha), flax, millet, potato starch, potato flour, quinoa, sorghum, soy, tapioca, and teff.

♦ Pasta made from rice, corn, buckwheat, quinoa, or any other gluten free grain; rice sticks and mung bean noodles. Some noodles are made with a percentage of wheat flour such as soba buckwheat noodles – read the ingredients carefully.

♦ Miscellaneous Ingredients. Annatto; citric, malic, and lactic acids; glucose syrup; guar gum; lecithin; maltodextrin (a corn derivative, unrelated to barley malt); plain spices; sucrose, dextrose, and lactose (if tolerant); baking soda, and cream of tartar; pure vanilla extract; active dry yeast; Xanthan gum

May Not Be Gluten Free...

♦ Deli or luncheon meats, frozen hamburgers or meatloaf, hot dogs or sausage, imitation crabmeat, vegetarian meat substitutes

♦ Tofu and seasoned tofu, tempeh may have wheat or barley ingredients.

♦ Seasoned shredded cheese, flavored yogurts

♦ Baked beans, seasoned canned beans, seasoned canned vegetables and tomatoes

♦ Seasoned or flavored rice mixes, nacho cheese sauces, flavored chips or corn chips, flavored nuts and soy nuts, licorice and candy, icings and frostings, chocolates, candy bars

- Soy sauce, mustards, salad dressings, specialty sauces and marinades

- Cooking sprays and butter flavored oils

- Flavored teas and coffee mixes, beer

- Oats are technically gluten free, but may be contaminated with other grains. If tolerant of oats, choose those designated as gluten free.

- Baking powder may contain wheat starch.

- Pharmaceuticals, lipsticks and cosmetics.

Just say NO...

- Wheat, and anything with wheat in its name except buckwheat (a misnomer, it is gluten free), and any form of wheat, such as bulgur, bread flour, cake flour, couscous, durum, einkorn, emmer, farina, faro, kamut, matzo, semolina, spelt, triticale, and wheat bran.

- Bread, pizza, hamburg or hotdog buns, cookies, crackers, pretzels, and other bakery items made from wheat, barley, or rye flour.

- Pasta or noodles made from wheat or spelt.

- Breakfast cereals, except those marked gluten free. (Corn flakes or rice crisps may contain malt flavoring, which is made from barley).

- Foods containing modified wheat starch, hydrolyzed wheat protein, malt flavoring, malt syrup, malt extract, and malt vinegar.

- Meats, poultry, seafood, or vegetables that have been breaded or floured, or are served with a sauce or gravy thickened with wheat flour or marinated in a mixture that contains soy sauce, tamari or teriyaki sauce. This includes most cafeteria entrees, frozen meals, fast foods, snack foods and deli take-out items. Beware of processed cold cuts at the deli area.

- Canned soups, and chicken, beef, and vegetable broths containing flour or hydrolyzed wheat protein, barley, or pasta.

- Beer (brewed from barley), alcoholic cooler beverages

For a complete and up-to-date ingredient lists, please refer to the extensive listings at www.celiac.com , or one of the gluten free brand name product services or books.

If in doubt, always contact directly the manufacturer of the food by phone or website.

About the Author

Joanne L. Bradley has extensive culinary experience gathered over 30 years in the foodservice industry. Starting out as a professional chef for 16 years, she then changed tracks and dedicated her career to making a difference in the college and university food service sector. Diagnosed with gluten and dairy intolerance while a University Food Service Director, she has since concentrated on gluten free culinary education.

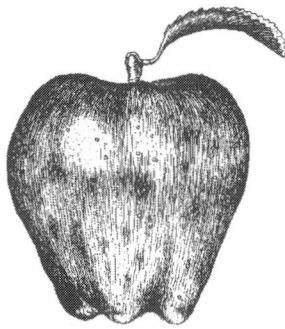

Gluten Free College Student Cookbook

About Gluten Free Success Publications...

Practical, real life knowledge about staying gluten free in unique life situations. That is our pledge to you, the gluten free reader and cook. We focus on providing quick and easy cooking instruction to speed you on your way to life beyond the kitchen.

For more information about our publications please visit...

www.GfCfSuccess.com

Gluten Free College Student Cookbook

Made in the USA
Lexington, KY
07 December 2010